Diabetic Meal Prep for Beginners

Type 1 Diabetes

The Ultimate Nutritional Guide With Three Healthy 4-Week Meal Plans And Shopping List. Use The Best Foods To Manage And Reverse Your Condition Now

Kate Green

Table of Contents

Introduction..**11**

What Is Diabetes? 11

How to Manage Diabetes?.....................................11

What Foods Should Be in a Diabetic Diet Plan?.......12

Chapter 1. What Do We Mean by Type 1 Diabetes? **14**

The Discovery of Insulin 14

Diabetes 15

Causes of Diabetes and Risk Factors 16

Signs and Symptoms of Diabetes 17

What Is Type 1 Diabetes? 17

How to Prevent Type 1 Diabetes?..........................19

    Diagnosis..*19*

    Treatments *19*

Chapter 2. Foods to Avoid...................................**21**

Sugars 21

High Fat Dairy Products 22

Saturated Animal Fats...22

High Carb Vegetables 22

Cholesterol Rich ingredients 23

High Sodium Products 23

Sugary Drinks...23

Sugar Syrups and Toppings 24

Sweet Chocolate and candies................................24

Alcohol...24

Chapter 3. Foods to Prefer..................................**25**

Diabetic Diet...25

What to Have on a Diabetic Diet 25

   Vegetables 25

   Meat 26

   Fruits 26

   Nuts and Seeds 27

   Grains 28

   Fats 28

   Diary 29

   Sugar Alternatives 29

Chapter 4. Benefits of Planning **31**

How to Manage Type 1 Diabetes? 31

   Get the Right Amount of Sleep 31

   Exercise 31

   Observe a Balanced Diet 32

Diabetic Meal Plans 32

6 Characteristics of a Diabetic Diet 32

How to Calculate Your Daily Carbohydrate, Protein, and Fat
Requirements (5 Steps) 34

Converting Grams to Calories 35

Getting Macronutrients from the Right Source 35

Distributing your Daily Calorie Needs 36

Recommended Schedule of Meals 36

Step by Step Guide to Distributing your Calories to Each Meal 38

What If the Amounts in Your Tabulation Are Too Low, Or Too High,
Compared to the Ideal Distribution? 39

Chapter 5. How to Make a Planning **40**

The Basics of Meal Prep 40

The Foods to Choose at the Store 40

Stocking Your Kitchen 42

How to Meal Plan 44

Chapter 6. Smart Ideas and Advice for Planning 46

Eating Refined Carbohydrates 46

Not Eating Whole Fruits 47

Not Keeping Track of Liquid Calories 47

Not Eating Enough Fiber-Rich Foods 47

Forgetting to Check Label for Ingredients 48

Eating Too Many Carbs 48

Eating Without Any Planning 48

Consuming Carb-Loaded Beverages 49

Skipping Dinner 49

Eating Too Much in Any Part of the Day 49

Craving for White Foods 50

Not Combining Carb and Protein 50

Missing Out on the Fiber Content 51

Focusing on Drinks than on Whole Foods 51

Eating Processed Meats and Making the Worst Choices for Breakfast
.... 51

Consuming High-Sugar Foods 51

Consuming Food That Spikes Your Blood Sugar Levels 52

Chapter 7. Week 1 Meal Plan: Healthy and Omnivorous and Weekly Shopping List 54

Breakfast 54

   1.   Cinnamon Overnight Oats 54

   2. Ham and Cheese English Muffin Melt 55

Snack 56

   3.   Garlic Kale Chips 56

Lunch 57

   4.   Egg Salad Wraps 57

   5.   Pizza Stuffed Pita.. 58

Snack 59

   6.   Caprese Skewers 59

Dinner.. 60

   7.   Minestrone 60

   8.   Zoodles with Pea Pesto 62

Chapter 8. Week 2 Meal Plan: Healthy and Omnivorous and Weekly Shopping List 63

Breakfast 63

   9.   Pumpkin Walnut Smoothie Bowl.............................. 63

   10.   Avocado Toast with Tomato and Cottage Cheese 64

Snack 65

   11.   Turkey Roll-Ups with Veggie Cream Cheese 65

Lunch 66

   12.   Almond Butter Apple Pita Pockets.................................... 66

   13.   Mason Jar Pear, Walnut, and Spinach Salad 66

Snacks 68

   14.   Baked Parmesan Crisps.. 68

Dinner.. 69

   15.   Shrimp Peri-Peri.. 69

   16.   Halibut with Lime and Cilantro 70

Chapter 9. Week 3 Meal Plan: Healthy and Omnivorous and Weekly Shopping List 71

Breakfast 71

   17.   Nutty Steel-cut Oatmeal with Blueberries.......................... 71

   18.   Quinoa Waffles 73

Snack 74

19.   Garlicky Hummus *74*

Lunch 75

20.   Mediterranean Steak Sandwiches *75*

21.   Chicken and Roasted Vegetable Wraps *77*

Snack 78

22.   Pesto Veggie Pizza *78*

Dinner 80

23.   Pork Chop Diane *80*

24.   Autumn Pork Chops with Red Cabbage and Apples *81*

Chapter 10. Week 4 Meal Plan: Healthy and Omnivorous and Weekly Shopping List 82

Breakfast 82

25.   Toasty Oatmeal Pancakes *82*

26.   Tomato-Herb Omelet *84*

Snack 86

27.   Apple Leather *86*

Lunch 88

28.   Almond-Crusted Salmon *88*

29.   Chicken & Veggie Bowl with Brown Rice *89*

Snack 91

30.   Simple Appetizer Meatballs *91*

Dinner 92

31.   Chipotle Chili Pork Chops *92*

32.   Orange-Marinated Pork Tenderloin *93*

Chapter 11. Week 1 Meal Plan: Vegetarian and Weekly Shopping List 94

Breakfast 94

33. Broccoli Omelet.. *94*

34. Wild Rice... *96*

Snack.. 97

35. French Bread Pizza.. *97*

Lunch... 98

36. Spinach Lasagna... *98*

37. Mushroom Soup with Sherry... *100*

Snack... 102

38. Spicy Bruschetta.. *102*

Dinner... 104

39. Vegetarian Chipotle Chili.. *104*

40. Crock Pot Veggies Soup.. *105*

Chapter 12. Week 2 Meal Plan: Vegetarian and Weekly Shopping List
.... **106**

Breakfast.. 106

41. Butternut Squash Risotto.. *106*

42. Slow "Roasted" Tomatoes... *108*

Snack... 110

43. Easy pizza for two *110*

Lunch... 111

44. Winter Vegetable Medley.. *111*

45. Classic Split Pea Soup *112*

Snack... 113

46. Bean Salad with Balsamic Vinaigrette............................... *113*

Dinner... 115

47. Squash Soup *115*

48. Easy Nacho Skillet Dinner.. *116*

Chapter 13. Week 3 Meal Plan: Vegetarian and Weekly Shopping List **117**

Breakfast 117

49. Coconut and Berry Smoothie.....................................*117*

50. Walnut and Oat Granola..*118*

Snack 120

51. Easy Cauliflower Hush Puppies.................................*120*

Lunch 122

52. Veggie Fajitas with Guacamole..................................*122*

53. Spaghetti Squash and Chickpea Bolognese.............*124*

Snack 125

54. Cauliflower Mash *125*

Dinner 127

55. Chimichurri Dumplings *127*

56. Redux Okra Callaloo *129*

Chapter 14. Week 4 Meal Plan: Vegetarian and Weekly Shopping List **130**

Breakfast 130

57. Coconut and Chia Pudding *130*

58. Cottage Pancakes *132*

Snack 133

59. Red Pepper, Goat Cheese, and Arugula Open-Faced Grilled Sandwich...*133*

Lunch 135

60. Beet, Goat Cheese, and Walnut Pesto with Zoodles...........*135*

61. Mushroom and Pesto Flatbread Pizza *137*

Snack 138

62. Cucumber, Tomato, and Avocado Salad...................*138*

Dinner.. 139

   63.   Black Bean Enchilada Skillet Casserole................................. *139*

   64.   Crispy Parmesan Cups with White Beans and Veggies....... *141*

Chapter 15. Bonus: Sauces and Desserts Recipes 143

   65.   Fruit-and-nut-stuffed Baked Apples...................................... *143*

   66.   Creamy Custard Sauce *145*

   67.   Orange and Pink Grapefruit Salad with Honey-rosemary Syrup
              ....*146*

   68.   Fruit-filled Meringues with Custard Sauce.......................... *147*

   69.   Frozen Yogurt.. *148*

   70.   Peach-blueberry Crostata... *149*

   71.   Creamy Goat Cheese—chive Dressing................................. *151*

   72.   Pecan Pie... *152*

   73.   Panna Cotta *154*

   74.   Tapioca Pudding *155*

   75.   Balsamic Vinaigrette *156*

Conclusion.. 157

Introduction

What Is Diabetes?

Diabetes mellitus is a condition in which a person's blood glucose (blood sugar) levels are too high. There are two types of diabetes: Type 1 and Type 2.

Type 1 Diabetes is often referred to as juvenile diabetes. It usually comes on suddenly in children, teenagers, and young adults and is not linked to being overweight. It is often, though not always, diagnosed when a person has a high blood glucose level. This type of diabetes is not preventable and treatment requires insulin injections.

Type 2 Diabetes generally starts slowly and builds over time. It used to be called adult-onset diabetes.

Diabetes has been known to affect many persons worldwide. According to a study, in 2015, about 28.1 million adults and nearly 586,000 children had diabetes. This is 2.8% of the U.S. population. The CDC also says another 86.4 million adults and 8.6 million children, or about 10.6% of the U.S. population, has prediabetes.

How to Manage Diabetes?

It is very important for persons with diabetes to have a doctor who can advise them on how to care for their condition. Persons with diabetes can control their blood glucose levels by taking medications, watching what they eat, and being physically active. When someone is diagnosed with diabetes, particularly Type 2 Diabetes, they are immediately advised to:

- Start on a healthy diet and get a lot of exercises.
- Know their target blood glucose levels and keep these levels within the blood.
- Get their blood glucose levels tested regularly. This will allow for good self-regulation of your blood glucose levels, and it will help your body become more efficient at managing glucose levels on its own.

It is important to have a healthy diet for diabetics and they need to pay extra attention to it. Unhealthy food is rich in both fat and carbohydrates and unhealthy eaters tend to eat a low fiber diet. Trans-fats, cholesterol, saturated fats, all can promote insulin resistance, boosting blood glucose levels.

What Foods Should Be in a Diabetic Diet Plan?

As diabetics, the diet plan should be properly supplemented with the right types and amounts of foods and some activities that can help you be healthy. There are several foods that are recommended to take in like green vegetables, juices, whole grains, lean meats, and fruits. We should consume the recommended amount of food if we are diabetics.

A diabetic diet plan is also important. People with diabetes often have to take insulin to control their blood glucose levels, so it is important to understand how insulin interacts with food. This interaction between certain foods (carbohydrates) and insulin can make it harder for the body to control blood glucose levels.

Lifestyle change. It can be hard for you to adapt to this change, but it is the only way that you would be able to fit dietary requirements that, hopefully, you can retain for the rest of your life.

As you start this journey on diabetic meal preparation, you are committing to a healthier lifestyle and sticking with it for the rest of your life. The lifestyle changes that people with diabetes have to undergo is not a joke, they call it a lifestyle change because it means you have to undergo permanent changes for the rest of your life.

Chapter 1. What Do We Mean by Type 1 Diabetes?

The Discovery of Insulin

The rapid growth of biological knowledge into the twentieth century, unfortunately, did not see as many improvements in the field of diabetes therapy. The future remained rather dark for those unfortunate insulin-dependent diabetes patients. In fact, in the first twenty years of this century, they had to face a short existence made up of suffering, not quite different from that described by Areteo, comparable to the prognosis for an advanced malignant neoplasm today. Those patients who decided to seek treatment were subjected to extremely strict diets which prolonged survival, and therefore suffering, only for a few months. However, several researchers were actively working on the discovery of the hypothetical insulin. One of them, Georg Sulzer, had even tested a pancreatic extract on humans, obtaining a patent for its preparation in America. However, these early preparations were of low and variable efficacy and often highly toxic, and none were ever actually useful in the treatment of the disease.

However, on January 23, 1922, a pancreatic extract prepared by Collip brought the blood sugar of a patient who was dying of diabetes back to normal, eliminated glycosuria and ketonuria, and thus represented the beginning of the use of insulin in the treatment of diabetes mellitus. Collip had developed an extraction technique capable of removing toxic contaminants from previously prepared crude pancreatic extracts and was able to effectively isolate the active ingredient. Since then, the group called the extract, at Macleod's suggestion, insulin, a name derived from the Latin root for pancreatic islets. Collip's technique was rudimentary and sometimes ineffective, and the team's problems with insulin production developed commercially usable extraction techniques based on isoelectric precipitation. By October 1923, insulin was widely available in North America and Europe. All this was possible thanks to the University of Toronto and its financiers who contributed decisively to the discovery by providing the group with all that, at the time, were cutting-edge materials and technologies and a significant number of experimental animals.

Diabetes

Diabetes is a chronic disease characterized by an increase in blood sugar i.e. the concentration of sugar in the blood that the body is unable to maintain within normal limits.

Hyperglycemia occurs when blood glucose exceeds 100mg/dl fasting or 140 mg/dl two hours after a meal. This condition may depend on a defect in function or a deficit in the production of insulin, the hormone secreted by the pancreas, used for the metabolism of sugars and other components of food to be transformed into energy for the whole organism (such as petrol for the engine).

When blood glucose levels are twice equal to or greater than 126mg/dl, diabetes is diagnosed: high blood glucose levels—if not treated—over time lead to chronic complications with damage to the kidneys, retina, nerves peripheral and cardiovascular system (heart and arteries).

Causes of Diabetes and Risk Factors

Although some of the causes are completely unclear, even trivial viral infections are recognized, which can attack and destroy insulin-producing cells in the pancreas, such as:

- Measles.
- Cytomegalovirus.
- Epstein-Barr.
- Coxsackievirus.

For Type 2 Diabetes, however, the main risk factors are:

- Overweight and obesity.
- Genetic factors: family history increases the risk of developing type 2 diabetes.
- Ethnicity: the highest number of cases is recorded in the populations of sub-Saharan Africa and the middle east and north Africa.
- Environmental factors are especially related to incorrect lifestyles (sedentary lifestyle and obesity).
- Gestational diabetes, which is diabetes that occurs during pregnancy.
- Age: type 2 diabetes increases with increasing age, especially above the age of 65.
- Diet high in fat that promotes obesity.

16

- Alcohol consumption.
- Sedentary lifestyle.

Signs and Symptoms of Diabetes

Symptoms of the disease, which depend on blood sugar levels, are:

- Polyuria, i.e. The high amount of urine production even during the night (nocturia).
- An intense feeling of thirst (polydipsia).
- Polyphagia (intense hunger).
- The body's need to replenish fluids and severe dehydration (dry mucous membranes).
- Feeling tired (asthenia).
- Weight loss.
- Frequent infections.
- Blurred vision.

In Type 1 Diabetes they manifest rapidly and with great intensity. In Type 2 Diabetes, on the other hand, symptoms are less evident, develop much slower, and may go unnoticed for months or years. Diagnosis often occurs by chance, on the occasion of tests done for any reason: the finding of a glycemia greater than 126 mg/dl allows the diagnosis of Type 2 diabetes, which must be confirmed with a second dosage of glycemia and HbA1c.

What Is Type 1 Diabetes?

Type 1 diabetes undergoes the destruction of the beta-cells in the pancreas that can produce insulin. It affects approximately 3-5% of people with diabetes and usually occurs in childhood or adolescence, but can also occur in adults. Type 1 diabetes is therefore characterized by beta-cell destruction, on an autoimmune or idiopathic basis, which leads to absolute insulin deficiency.

It is now known that at the base of the disease there is a "sabotage" by the immune system against the cells that produce insulin: the disease manifests itself in fact with the presence in the blood antibodies directed against antigens present in the cells that produce insulin. It is, for this reason, that type 1 diabetes is classified among the so-called "autoimmune" diseases, characterized by a reaction of the immune system against the organism itself. The damage that the immune system induces against the cells that produce insulin is believed it may be linked to hereditary factors and/or environmental factors (including diet, lifestyle, contact with specific viruses).

In type 1 diabetes, symptoms tend to arise more quickly and more severely than in type 2 diabetes. Symptoms related manifest themselves with:

- Fatigue.
- Increased thirst (polydipsia).
- Increased urine output (polyuria).
- Unwanted weight loss despite hyperphagia (increased appetite).
- Malaise.
- Abdominal pain.

In the most serious cases, mental confusion and loss of consciousness may also occur. The major complications deriving from diabetes can cause the patient even significant damage to the neurological, renal, ocular, and cardio-cerebrovascular levels.

How to Prevent Type 1 Diabetes?

Type 1 Diabetes cannot currently be prevented: no preventive strategy has so far proved effective. However, preventive action for conditions like Type 2 Diabetes which are believed to help prevent Type 1 Diabetes includes these:

- Prefer foods low in fat and calories, consume fruit and vegetables in abundance.
- Engage in moderate aerobic physical activity for at least 20 to 30 minutes per day (or 150 minutes per week).
- Keeping fit weight, avoiding conditions like overweight, and obesity.

Diagnosis

A blood test is required to diagnose diabetes. For the diagnosis of diabetes, a fasting glucose value greater than 126mg/dl confirmed on at least two different days is sufficient.

Treatments

To treat Type 1 Diabetes, the only therapy available is the intake of insulin, by means of subcutaneous injections. Thanks to this therapy and the correct lifestyle, most patients manage to lead a normal life and prevent the onset of long-term complications. It becomes essential for the adequate treatment of Type 1 Diabetes to access specialized centers where

19

there is an interaction between the various specialists (diabetologists, ophthalmologists, nephrologists, cardiologists), the use of advanced technologies (insulin pumps and Holter type glycemic monitoring), new drugs (innovative insulins) associated with indispensable educational techniques (CHO counting, physical activity, diet).

Chapter 2. Foods to Avoid

Knowing a general scheme of diet helps a lot, but it is equally important to be well familiar with the items which have to be avoided. With this list, you can make your diet a hundred% sugar-free. There are many other food items which can cause some harm to a diabetic patient as the sugars do. So, let's discuss them in some detail here.

Sugars

Sugar is a big NO-GO for a diabetic diet. Once you are diabetic, you would need to say goodbye to all the natural sweeteners which are loaded with carbohydrates. They contain polysaccharides which readily break into glucose after getting into our body. And the list does not only include table sugars but other items like honey and molasses should also be avoided.

1. White sugar
2. Brown sugar
3. Confectionary sugar
4. Honey
5. Molasses
6. Granulated sugar

It is not easy to suddenly stop using sugar. Your mind and your body, will not accept the abrupt change. It is recommended to go for a gradual change. It means start substituting it with low carb substitutes in a small amount, day by day.

High Fat Dairy Products

Once you are diabetic, you may get susceptible to a number of other fatal diseases including cardiovascular ones. That is why experts strictly recommend avoiding high-fat food products, especially dairy items. The high amount of fat can make your body insulin resistant. So even when you take insulin, it won't be of any use as the body will not work on it.

Saturated Animal Fats

Saturated animal fats are not good for anyone, whether diabetic or normal. So, better avoid using them in general. Whenever you are cooking meat, try to trim off all the excess fat. Cooking oils made out of these saturated fats should be avoided. Keep yourself away from any of the animal origin fats.

High Carb Vegetables

As discussed above, vegetables with more starch are not suitable for diabetes. These veggies can increase the carbohydrate levels of food. So, omit these from the recipes and enjoy the rest of the less starchy vegetables. Some of the high carb vegetables are:

1. Potatoes
2. Sweet potatoes
3. Yams etc.

Cholesterol Rich ingredients

Bad cholesterol or High-density Lipoprotein has the tendency to deposit in different parts of the body and obstructs the flow of blood and the regulation of hormones. That is why food items having high bad cholesterol are not good for diabetes. Such items should be replaced with the ones with low cholesterol.

High Sodium Products

Sodium is related to hypertension and blood pressure. Since diabetes is already the result of a hormonal imbalance in the body, in the presence of excess sodium—another imbalance—a fluid imbalance may occur which a diabetic body cannot tolerate. It adds up to already present complications of the disease. So, avoid using food items with a high amount of sodium. Mainly store packed items, processed foods, and salt all contain sodium, and one should avoid them all. Use only the 'Unsalted' variety of food products, whether it's butter, margarine, nuts, or other items.

Sugary Drinks

Cola drinks or other similar beverages are filled with sugars. If you had seen different video presentations showing the amount of the sugars present in a single bottle of soda, you would know how dangerous those are for diabetic patients. They can drastically increase the amount of blood glucose level within 30 minutes of drinking. Fortunately, there are many sugar-free varieties available in the drinks which are suitable for diabetic patients.

Sugar Syrups and Toppings

A number of syrups available in the markets are made out of nothing but sugar. Maple syrup is one good example. For a diabetic diet, the patient should avoid such sugary syrups and also stay away from the sugar-rich toppings available in the stores. If you want to use them at all, trust yourself and prepare them at home with a sugar-free recipe.

Sweet Chocolate and candies

For diabetic patients, sugar-free chocolates or candies are the best way out. Other processed chocolate bars and candies are extremely damaging to their health, and all of these should be avoided. You can try and prepare healthy bars and candies at home with sugar-free recipes.

Alcohol

Alcohol has the tendency to reduce the rate of our metabolism and take away our appetite, which can render a diabetic patient into a very life-threatening condition. Alcohol in a very small amount cannot harm the patient, but the regular or constant intake of alcohol is bad for health and glucose levels.

Chapter 3. Foods to Prefer

Diabetic Diet

Treatment through the dietary approach is considered the most effective and logical today. Many of the fatal health conditions are now treated only with a well-oriented health diet plan. The same is true for diabetes. With few adjustments in the routine menu, a patient can maintain his glucose levels without the use of medicines. To make this idea work, we need to cut down the direct or high sources of glucose in the food. Here is the complete list of the items which can be taken on a diabetes-friendly diet.

What to Have on a Diabetic Diet

Vegetables

Fresh vegetables never cause harm to anyone. So, adding a meal full of vegetables is the best shot for all diabetic patients. But not all vegetables contain the same amount of macronutrients. Some vegetables contain a high amount of carbohydrates, so those are not suitable for a diabetic diet. We need to use vegetables which contain a low amount of carbohydrates.

1. Cauliflower
2. Spinach
3. Tomatoes
4. Broccoli
5. Lemons

6. Artichoke
7. Garlic
8. Asparagus
9. Spring onions
10. Onions
11. Ginger etc.

Meat

Meat is not on the red list for the diabetic diet. It is fine to have some meat every now and then for diabetic patients. However certain meat types are better than others. For instance, red meat is not a preferable option for such patients. They should consume white meat more often whether it's seafood or poultry. Healthy options in meat are:

1. All fish, i.e., salmon, halibut, trout, cod, sardine, etc.
2. Scallops
3. Mussels
4. Shrimp
5. Oysters etc.

Fruits

Not all fruits are good for diabetes. To know if the fruit is suitable for this diet, it is important to note its sugar content. Some fruits contain a high amount of sugars in the form of sucrose and fructose, and those should be readily avoided. Here is the list of popularly used fruits which can be taken on the diabetic diet:

1. Peaches
2. Nectarines
3. Avocados
4. Apples
5. Berries
6. Grapefruit
7. Kiwi Fruit
8. Bananas
9. Cherries
10. Grapes
11. Orange
12. Pears
13. Plums
14. Strawberries

Nuts and Seeds

Nuts and seeds are perhaps the most enriched edibles, and they contain such a mix of macronutrients which can never harm anyone. So diabetic patients can take the nuts and seeds in their diet without any fear of a glucose spike.

1. Pistachios
2. Sunflower seeds
3. Walnuts
4. Peanuts
5. Pecans
6. Pumpkin seeds

7. Almonds

8. Sesame seeds etc.

Grains

Diabetic patients should also be selective while choosing the right grains for their diet. The idea is to keep the amount of starch as minimum as possible. That is why you won't see any white rice in the list rather it is replaced with more fibrous brown rice.

1. Quinoa

2. Oats

3. Multigrain

4. Whole grains

5. Brown rice

6. Millet

7. Barley

8. Sorghum

9. Tapioca

Fats

Fat intake is the most debated topic as far as the diabetic diet is concerned. As there are diets like ketogenic, which are loaded with fats and still proved effective for diabetic patients. The key is the absence of carbohydrates. In any other situation, the fats are as harmful to diabetics as any normal person. Switching to unsaturated fats is a better option.

1. Sesame oil

2. Olive oil

3. Canola oil

4. Grapeseed oil

5. Other vegetable oils

6. Fats extracted from plant sources.

Diary

Any dairy product which directly or indirectly causes a glucose rise in the blood should not be taken on this diet. other than those, all products are good to use. These items include:

1. Skimmed milk

2. Low-fat cheese

3. Eggs

4. Yogurt

5. Trans fat-free margarine or butter

Sugar Alternatives

Since ordinary sugars or sweeteners are strictly forbidden on a diabetic diet. There are artificial varieties that can add sweetness without raising the level of carbohydrates in the meal. These substitutes are:

1. Stevia

2. Xylitol

3. Natvia

4. Swerve

5. Monk fruit

6. Erythritol

Make sure to substitute them with extra care. The sweetness of each sweetener is entirely different from the table sugar, so add each in accordance with the intensity of their flavor. Stevia is the sweetest of them, and it should be used with more care. In place of 1 cup of sugar, a teaspoon of stevia is enough. All other sweeteners are more or less similar to sugar in their intensity of sweetness.

Chapter 4. Benefits of Planning

How to Manage Type 1 Diabetes?

Aside from insulin injections, there are certain things a type 1 diabetic needs to amend in their lifestyle, to avoid complications. Here are a few dos and don'ts.

Get the Right Amount of Sleep

The correct amount of sleep is important for everyone. However, if a Type 1 diabetic does not get the correct amount of sleep, complications can arise.

It needs to be "the correct amount of sleep." A diabetic person should not sleep for too long a period, as it increases the risk of hypoglycemia. Blood sugar levels tend to drop when the body is at rest.

If a person does not get enough sleep, they may suffer from hyperglycemia (high blood sugar), as the blood circulates faster when a person is awake.

Exercise

This may be a difficult task for a type I diabetic as they can easily tire, but it is necessary. Type 1 diabetics should exercise more if they want to lower the amount of insulin they require. Physical activity helps to process carbohydrates or glucose, so the more a person exercises, the less insulin they will require. Exercise also helps improve your body's sensitivity to insulin, as a person burns calories doing physical activity.

Observe a Balanced Diet

Since a type 1 diabetic cannot process glucose effectively, it is only logical that they should lower their sugar intake. Experts agree that regardless of the nature of the person's diet, they should be mindful of their carbohydrates and sugar intake.

It is recommended that diabetics eat small meals, every 2 to 3 hours, instead of eating large meals every 4 to 6 hours. This way, the glucose consumed is at a constant level. This limits the chance of experiencing hypoglycemic or hyperglycemic attacks.

Diabetic Meal Plans

Many nutritionists believe the diet followed by diabetics is a good diet for everyone. Anyone who follows it lowers their risk of developing diabetes and other health conditions.

6 Characteristics of a Diabetic Diet

Experts say that the ideal diabetic diet has the following characteristics:

- It is low in calories. Diabetics should eat a low-calorie diet, as opposed to a low carbohydrate diet. Lowering calories means you lower the actual amount of carbohydrate and fat you need to burn.

  Low-carbohydrate and low-fat diets may not work for diabetics, as they may then increase proteins in the digestive tract and the bloodstream to a dangerous level. Diabetic people should not consume a large amount of protein, as it may increase their risk of neuropathy and other complications. If the amount of fat and carbs, in the diet, is significantly decreased, while the amount of protein remains at a proportionate level, the diabetic may suffer from malnutrition. Thus, the solution is to lower the overall calorie intake.

- The number of carbohydrates should not be less than 45%, but no more than 60% of the total calorie intake each day.

- For pregnant and breastfeeding women, the amount should not be less than 50%.

- The amount of protein should not exceed 1 gram, for every 0.45kg of his/her ideal weight, and no lower than 0.4 grams.

- The amount of fat in a diabetic's diet should not be more than 25% of the amount of the ideal total calorie allowance for the day.

- Their diet should have less fried and processed food.

Fried and processed foods are high in unhealthy fat and refined carbohydrates. They increase the level of glucose in the blood, blocking insulin receptors and increasing cravings for sweet and greasy food.

Foods that retain their natural flavor are usually high in fiber and low in sugar. Fiber aids digestion and helps "choose" which nutrients are absorbed, or not, by the body.

How to Calculate Your Daily Carbohydrate, Protein, and Fat Requirements (5 Steps)

Using the characteristics of a diabetic diet, we can calculate the ideal amount of carbohydrates, proteins, and fat needed for a balanced diet. Here is a step-by-step approach to balancing the type of food in the diet.

Step 1: Know your ideal weight.

Step 2: Choose your ideal total calorie intake for the day.

Step 3: Calculate how much protein you need in calories.

Since proteins must be proportional to your weight, it is better to calculate this first. Multiply your ideal weight by an amount within 0.4 to 1 gram per pound. Multiply the result by four.

Step 4: Calculate the number of carbohydrates.

The ideal amount is usually somewhere between 45-60%. It should be proportional to the degree of the person's physical activity. If they are very active, they could consume as much as 60%.

Step 5: Allocate the remaining amount to fat.

This should not exceed 25%. The remaining number of calories can be allocated to fat. However, if the level of fat exceeds 25% of the total calorie intake, then the ideal total calorie intake should be lowered.

For children under seventeen years of age, the amount of fat can be increased to 30%.

Converting Grams to Calories

Most food manufacturers on the market list their product facts using grams. It is enforced by states, but also a marketing strategy. The number of grams is smaller than the number of calories. If a consumer sees the product only has 15 grams of fat, he might not be too worried. However, if they see the product contains 135 calories from fat, they might think twice.

Ignoring these totals is not an option for diabetics. They need to be more vigilant in knowing how many grams/calories they consume each day. They must convert the weight in grams to calories. Knowing this helps them to arrange the correct meal plan for the whole day.

Some might think that this is too complex. However, diabetics do not always have to calculate the calorie value for each food. Diabetic associations often supply dietary guides that include conversions.

If you cannot find a manual, you can do it using the table below:

1. 1 gram of carbohydrate is the equivalent of 4 calories.
2. 1 gram of protein is equivalent to 4 calories.
3. 1 gram of fat is the equivalent of 9 calories.

Getting Macronutrients from the Right Source

Another vital aspect of a diabetic plan is choosing the source of your food. A diabetic may be eating the correct amount of protein, carbohydrates, and fats, but if they are coming from a bad source, his/her diet will not be healthy.

According to nutritionists, diabetics should source their carbohydrates, fat, and protein from natural and unrefined foods.

Processed foods break down into synthetic chemicals that may be harmful to the body even though they may contain the same amount of nutrient

Distributing your Daily Calorie Needs

Knowing how many grams you need and the type of food to fulfill your daily calorie needs is only one side of the equation. The second part of planning is dividing your daily calorie needs among your meals.

One suggested approach is that you reduce the size of your meals as nighttime approaches. Specifically, you should:

- Eat a heavier Breakfast;
- Eat a moderate lunch;
- Eat a light dinner/supper.

However, some believe this rule is not acceptable for all diabetics; and in fact, many experts state this approach is only suitable for prediabetics. It is not advisable for type 1 diabetics, as they may suffer from hypoglycemia while they sleep, due to the lack of carbohydrates.

Recommended Schedule of Meals

A more acceptable schedule is eating five small meals a day, with sufficient intervals between meals. Below is one recommended schedule of meals for a diabetic.

- **Breakfast should not be more than twelve hours after supper.**

Some dieticians may disagree with this. Blood sugar levels could drop to dangerous levels if the person fasts for more than 10 hours. However, some doctors and experts still recommend a twelve-hour interval between supper and Breakfast.

A diabetic is advised to drink a glass of milk before bedtime, to avoid hypoglycemia.

- **Snacks should be between two to three hours after meals (Breakfast and Lunch).**

Snacks should not be skipped, even if the diabetic does not feel hungry.

Diabetics often complain of hunger two to three hours after eating a meal, when in fact, they are not hungry. It is the body sending a misleading signal to the brain and other organs. If the diabetic ignores these signals, the body wants to defend itself and the organs try to protect themselves from hunger by conserving energy. Diabetic complications may arise as a result of this. So, doctors suggest eating a small amount of food, regularly. This helps produce enzymes that convince the body it is not hungry.

- **Lunch should not be more than 6 hours after Breakfast.**

Diabetics should, on no account, skip lunch, especially type 1 diabetic. Diabetics need a regular intake of carbohydrates to maintain their blood sugar level. Skipping lunch or any meals may trigger ketoacidosis.

- **Dinner/Supper should be more than 6 hours, but not more than 10 hours from lunch.**

Supper is just as important as Breakfast, for diabetics. The body needs a store of carbohydrates and fat, for the body to process while it is asleep. If there is nothing to process, it can trigger hypoglycemia and in some cases for type 1 diabetic, ketoacidosis.

Step by Step Guide to Distributing your Calories to Each Meal

Here are the steps to help you allocate the number of calories for each meal:

- Divide your ideal daily calorie needs into four.

Though you need five meals a day, you only need to divide your total calorie needs into four because one portion is divided into two snack portions.

- Let's assume your ideal daily calorie needs are 1800. Then, each meal should be approximately 450 calories, with two snacks of 225 calories.
- Calculate how much carbohydrate, protein, and fat do you need for the day.
- List what you would like to eat for each meal. A diabetic diet does not limit your choice, but ideally, it needs to be healthy, unrefined, and within your daily calorie allowance.
- List the carbohydrate and fat and protein for each meal.

Tabulate everything. Compute the total of the calories, grams of fat, protein, and carbohydrates.

Compare the meal total planned with your ideal distribution. You need to check whether your meals fit within your ideal calorie distribution.

What If the Amounts in Your Tabulation Are Too Low, Or Too High, Compared to the Ideal Distribution?

The planned meal is too low from the ideal distribution if it falls below 1000 calories. It is too high if it exceeds 2500 calories.

Falling or exceeding your ideal calorie distribution for one or two days may not cause problems but, doing so on a regular basis often causes complications.

If your actual calorie intake is significantly lower, then the diet is not providing the correct nutrition your body requires. This could result in malnutrition, frequent weakness, and frequent hypoglycemia.

If it is significantly higher than the ideal calorie distribution, it will not control blood sugar levels and increase the risk of diabetic complications.

Chapter 5. How to Make a Planning

The Basics of Meal Prep

It is time for us first to look into the basics of being able to prep and plan your meals to help keep your diet on track. Being able to prep and plan your meals can help you greatly with making sure that you stay healthy and to ensure that your food is nourishing your body the right way. We are going to address topics such as how to choose healthy foods at the store and how you should be working to stock your kitchen. You will also see what goes into planning a diet, how you can determine what the right foods for your meal plan will be, and you will be introduced to meal prepping—the idea that you can create your meals and even start with parts of your meals in advance so that you can cut down the cooking time when it's time to eat.

The Foods to Choose at the Store

It's easy for you to think that you are making a good choice for your food, only to realize that the choice that you did make is actually not very practical or healthy at all. In particular, when we see all of these different foods that claim on their packaging that they are healthy or complete, we can run into a very simple problem—we buy things without actually knowing what is in them. However, you can avoid that problem just by learning what you should be looking for when you are shopping. Here are some tips when you are making your shopping plans:

- **Always read the nutrition label:** No matter what the front box says, make sure that you always take the time to figure out what is actually inside the foods that you pick up. Double-check how healthy the food that you are looking at actually is. Make sure that you check the label—and compare it to other options as well. Take the time to compare the ingredients and choose those that have the lowest amounts of sodium, unhealthy fats, and sugars.

- **Avoid tricky ingredients:** A lot of ingredients that are in your food are hidden under other names. You might not see sugar on the top three ingredients—but is high fructose corn syrup up there? Or any other of those ingredients? That ending is specific to sugars, and if you know that it is high in one of the other –those endings, you know that it is actually high in sugar, even if it doesn't say sugar

- **If fresh food isn't available, always choose frozen:** When you have to choose between no food and frozen food, you should choose the frozen. If you can't get frozen, choose canned, but make sure that you choose options that are lower in sodium and added sugars or syrups.

- **Opt for whole-grain ingredients:** when you go shopping; make sure that you choose those whole-grain options. Pasta, bread, crackers, and all sorts of other foods all come in whole-grain forms that will help you enjoy them without getting those high blood sugar spikes.

- **If you can't pronoz. the ingredients, avoid it:** Take a look at the ingredient names. Making sure that you eat mostly healthy whole

41

foods, also means making sure that you should actually recognize the names of what you are eating.

Stocking Your Kitchen

Of course, any good meal plan is only as good as the kitchen that it is cooked in, and that means that you need to make sure that you are giving yourself plenty of good foods that will keep you full for longer. Here are essential food items that you can keep in your kitchen at all times. Consider these the basics that you should keep constantly stocked on top of anything else that you may decide that you want to eat based on your meal plan.

Whole grains to keep on hand

- Whole wheat flours and oats
- Brown rice
- Whole wheat bread, cereals, and pasta
- Quinoa

Beans and legumes to keep on hand

- Variety of canned beans (red, pinto, garbanzo, etc.)
- Dried lentils and peas

Healthy fats to keep on hand

- No sugar added nut butter
- Olive oil
- Coconut oil
- Canola oil
- Avocado oil

Canned fruits and veggies to keep on hand

- Tomatoes (diced and sauced)
- Green beans
- Artichokes Fresh produce to keep on hand
- In-season produce
- Citrus fruits of choice
- Avocados
- Onions
- Sweet potatoes
- Spinach
- Kale
- Broccoli
- Zucchini
- Squash
- Tomatoes

Protein sources to keep on hand

- Canned salmon or tuna in water, not oil
- Chicken breast
- Fresh meats of choice
- Eggs

Snacks to keep on hand

- Whole-grain crackers (low-carb)
- Multi-grain chips
- Seeds and nuts (unsalted)

- Popcorn

Seasonings to keep on hand

- Garlic
- Herbs and spices to limit salt content

How to Meal Plan

Now consider that you will need to plan out your meals to make sure that you stick to the right tasks at hand. Making your shopping list and avoiding the frustration of figuring out what you are going to eat is all simplified with one simple task: Meal planning.

In meal planning, you make yourself a menu for the week. You make it so that you are able to find the meals that will work for you to make sure that you are eating foods that will be healthy, but also so that you don't unnecessarily buy foods that you don't actually need. To plan a meal plan, all you need to do, then, is write down what you will eat that week.

Breakfasts, lunches, dinners, and snacks should all be planned out. When you do that and make sure that you know what it is that you want to eat, you can then assemble your shopping list. When you have that shopping list, you buy only what you need, meaning that you save money and avoid waste!

Your meal plan should incorporate meals with similar ingredients so that you can either reuse the same bunch of ingredients, or it may contain leftovers intentionally to slow down how much you have to cook.

When you have your meal plan, you have a few simple benefits—you are able to meal prep, for example. You can make sure that you prepare ingredients in advance if it works better for your schedule. When you do this, you can make meals that might have a lot of prep actually work better during days that are actually quite busy. Say you want to eat enchiladas for dinner, for example, but you are going to be busy. The best way to make that work is to prep what you can before that. When you know what you will be eating, you know that you can prep the foods that you want in advance and know that you aren't just taking a shot in the dark.

Chapter 6. Smart Ideas and Advice for Planning

It is necessary to learn from your errors when you have diabetes. Some health issues, such as weight gain and elevated blood pressure, may also be reduced as a result. You should benefit from the flaws of other individuals, too. It could help you escape problems and accomplish the targets of your therapy.

Diabetes is a disorder marked by high amounts of blood sugar. It is one of the main metabolic diseases worldwide at present. By consuming a balanced diet and living a safe lifestyle, diabetes can be treated. It is claimed that trans-fats, refined, and excessively sugary diets raise blood sugar levels, so diabetics are also told to reduce them. They are even advised to avoid drinking and quit smoking. There are a number of things that diabetics should either consume or avoid if they want to lead a happy and healthy life that is free from any critical diabetic-related health issues. Listed below are the mistakes that a diabetic person must avoid, along with some healthy dietary recommendations:

Eating Refined Carbohydrates

It is time to phase out from your diet processed grains and goods and consume more whole foods such as whole grains, cereals, vegetables, etc. In the course of processing, finished grains are stripped of all their fibers and a lot of nutrients. Whole grains do not experience such extensive refining; their minerals are also not swept out. Brown rice, oatmeal, quinoa, millet, or amaranth are other whole grains you might check out. It is believed that all these grains and millets have a positive influence on the blood glucose level.

Not Eating Whole Fruits

Integrate a whole lot of seasonal fruits and vegetables in your diet. They are rich in fiber that helps to regulate your blood sugar levels. Get more of the whole fruit, if possible. Juicing fruits can deprive you of vital fibers. When essential fibers are extracted in the juicing process, the natural sugar content often becomes more concentrated.

Not Keeping Track of Liquid Calories

It's not enough to only keep track of the solid foods you consume. You must also be aware of the intake of drinks. It may be dangerous to the blood sugar levels to consume aerated foods, sodas, and iced-teas/coffee that are sugary. These beverages contain a lot of sugar and calories that must be stopped by the diabetics.

Not Eating Enough Fiber-Rich Foods

Ensure that the diet is rich with enough foods abundant in nutrients. To dissolve and digest, fiber requires a large amount. This helps the bloodstream to absorb sugar steadily, which maintains steady levels of blood sugar.

Forgetting to Check Label for Ingredients

Do not hesitate to search the label on all the ingredients while you are picking up anything from a store. Check for items in them that have sugar. Even tomato ketchup, sauces, and dressings are filled with extra sugar and may not be particularly prescribed for diabetics.

Eating Too Many Carbs

Carbs are not harmful to you, considering that you eat them in moderation and that you eat the best sort of carbs. However, it can potentially affect the blood sugar levels from eating so many sugars, which can lead to long-term medical conditions such as cardiovascular disease, obesity, and diabetes. Carbohydrate overload is a basic issue of diabetics. A half-cup serving of pasta contains 15 grams of carbohydrate. You probably eat more than ½ cup of pasta in your meals.

Eating Without Any Planning

The hectic schedules that we pursue have a detrimental effect on our consumption of food. For optimum diabetes treatment, meal prep is the most important thing. You must spare some time, at least once a week, to decide about the next week's menu. Based on your menu schedule, make your shopping list and stick to the list.

You won't get stuck running through a fast-food drive-thru or cooking up high-carbohydrate frozen meals if you go by your meal plan and stick to it.

Consuming Carb-Loaded Beverages

Milk, juices, soft pop, sports drinks, caffeine drinks, and energy drinks will all work toward the optimum glucose regulation activities. Although, you will often be told that plain water is the best for treating diabetes. It is free of calories and soothing. While making your fruit choices, you can pick cucumber, fresh mint, or lime.

Skipping Dinner

You had a very sumptuous lunch with your customer or friend. Moreover, the time comes for dinner or other meals, and you really aren't ready. What're you doing? Well, it will definitely have detrimental effects on glucose by missing out on the evening meal. Consider eating a sandwich on whole-grain bread. You may also eat an apple if you just are not hungry enough for dinner. With about 45 grams of carbohydrate, that will fuel your body.

You can get 45 grams of carbs even with 1 cup of yogurt mixed with 1 cup of berries and ½ banana. Don't go to bed without a meal, even though you've had a massive noon meal. And do not overeat at lunch next time; take ½ of it home for your evening dinner.

Eating Too Much in Any Part of the Day

It's the biggest meal of the day, typically. Almost all meals should be comparable in size and carbohydrate content for optimum glucose regulation. Scale your evening meal down if it's too heavy. Select the optimum amount of carbohydrate/starch to prepare your meals in the kitchen.

Craving for White Foods

You've undoubtedly read this before, that you should quit white foods. Although the purpose behind this clear declaration is usually positive in the beginning, it has some negative consequences. Foods like white rice, bread, and flour are not safe for consumption by people suffering from diabetes.

However, patients fear cauliflower, cottage cheese, onions, and turnips because they are white. There are white foods that are balanced. In short, be aware of the nutritional content of the foods that you drink.

Not Combining Carb and Protein

Perhaps you need to be aware of the kind of foods you consume, because if you only eat carbs then it can turn into sugar far faster than if you consume it with protein. So, make sure that to slow down the conversion process, you eat your carbs with some sort of protein.

Apple slices, sunflower seed butter, almond butter, and cashew butter are some of the popular foods that patients might consume. They taste much better, are good for diabetic people, and they often appear to contain limited "filler" ingredients. If you can, go organic. It will be much safer.

Missing Out on the Fiber Content

Breakfast also offers an excellent opportunity to consume some fiber, which is essential for diabetes because, without increasing your blood pressure, fiber fills you up. This may mean greater regulation of blood-sugar and fewer calories. Diabetic people, in their Breakfast, generally do not consume fiber, which is a major mistake because consuming 7 to 10 grams of fiber each morning is a great meal for diabetes.

Focusing on Drinks than on Whole Foods

While some people prefer Breakfast drinks, whole foods provide a much healthier option. Drinking juices is a common trend, but bear in mind that there are essential carbohydrates and calories in one big serving of juiced fruit. That means you can experience a spike in blood sugar and weight gain very often from juicing.

Eating Processed Meats and Making the Worst Choices for Breakfast

You don't add carbs to your diet with bacon, sausage, and ham, but they're not good protein options either. With little to no nutrients, poor Breakfast options include disproportionate calories. Keep away from snack bars, big whipped cream, and caramel coffee drinks, sweetened cereals, and pastries.

Consuming High-Sugar Foods

Consuming down doughnuts and coffee for the extra sugar and caffeine if you don't have a lot of time in the morning for nutritious Breakfast meals

51

is a mistake. For the next couple of hours, Breakfast can be a meal that gives the body energy. It ought to be a useful energy source, not just swift energy. You will get a brief sugar spike from a doughnut and coffee with sugar, but you will not have done your body any good, because it will wear off fast, potentially culminating in a blood-sugar collapse.

People with diabetes sometimes believe like their drugs can counterbalance the sugar they eat, so they don't try to limit calories, candy, and even desserts. For the ultimate diabetes treatment method, this may prove risky.

Consuming Food That Spikes Your Blood Sugar Levels

People tend to eat or consume food that is harmful to the effective management of diabetes. Given below are the foods that diabetics should exclude from their meals:

- Fruit juice
- Dried fruit
- Only fruit
- Starchy vegetables, for example, peas, winter squash, corn, and sweet potatoes
- Beans
- Peas
- Lentils
- Dairy products that are low in fat, for example, sweetened yogurt
- Bread(grain)
- Pasta

- Rice
- Cereal
- Oatmeal
- Crackers
- Pretzels
- Snack foods that have been processed, for example, potato chips, tortilla chips
- Fried foods, for example, doughnuts, and French fries
- Fried chicken
- Sweets, for example, candy, cake, ice cream, pie, pastries, and cookies
- Beverages that have been sweetened by mixing sugar, for example, soft drinks, energy drinks, sugar-sweetened coffee and tea, and drinks that are consumed by athletes
- Alcoholic beverages
- Processed meats
- Fatty red meat
- Poultry with skin
- Solid fats, for example, lard and butter
- Mixed drinks
- Flavored yogurt
- Flavored oatmeal
- Sugary condiments
- Dried fruit and fruit juice

Chapter 7. Week 1 Meal Plan: Healthy and Omnivorous and Weekly Shopping List

Breakfast

1. Cinnamon Overnight Oats

Preparation Time: 5 minutes, plus overnight to refrigerate

Cooking Time: 0 minutes

Servings: 2

Ingredients:

- ⅔ cup unsweetened almond milk
- ⅔ cup rolled oats
- ½ apple, cored and finely chopped
- 2 tablespoons chopped walnuts
- 1 teaspoon cinnamon
- Pinch sea salt

Directions:

1. In a single-serving container or mason jar, combine all of the ingredients and mix well.
2. Cover and refrigerate overnight.

Nutrition:

- Calories: 242 kcal
- Total Fat: 12g
- Saturated Fat: 1g
- Sodium: 97mg

- Carbohydrates: 30g
- Fiber: 6g
- Protein: 6g

2. Ham and Cheese English Muffin Melt

Preparation Time: 10 minutes

Cooking Time: 5 minutes

Servings: 2

Ingredients:

- 1 whole-grain English muffin, split and toasted
- 2 teaspoons Dijon mustard
- 2 slices tomato
- 4 thin slices deli ham
- ½ cup shredded Cheddar cheese
- 2 large eggs, fried (optional)

Directions:

1. Preheat the oven broiler on high.
2. Spread each toasted English muffin half with 1 teaspoon of mustard, and place them on a rimmed baking sheet, cut-side up.
3. Top each with a tomato slice and 2 slices of ham. Sprinkle each with half of the cheese.
4. Broil in the preheated oven until the cheese melts, 2 to 3 minutes.
5. Serve immediately, topped with a fried egg, if desired.

Nutrition:

- Calories: 234 kcal
- Total Fat: 13g
- Saturated Fat: 7g
- Sodium: 834mg
- Carbohydrates: 16g
- Fiber: 3g
- Protein: 16g

Snack

3. Garlic Kale Chips

Preparation Time: 5 minutes

Cooking Time: 15 minutes

Servings: 2

Ingredients:

- 1 (16 oz.) bunch kale, trimmed and cut into 2-inch pieces
- 2 tablespoons extra-virgin olive oil
- 1 teaspoon sea salt
- ½ teaspoon garlic powder
- Pinch cayenne (optional, to taste)

Directions:

1. Preheat the oven to 350°F. Line two baking sheets with parchment paper.
2. Wash the kale and pat it completely dry.
3. In a large bowl, toss the kale with the olive oil, sea salt, garlic powder, and cayenne, if using.
4. Spread the kale in a single layer on the prepared baking sheets.
5. Bake until crisp, 12 to 15 minutes, rotating the sheets once.

Nutrition:

- Calories: 231 kcal
- Total Fat: 15g
- Saturated Fat: 2g
- Sodium: 678mg
- Carbohydrates: 20g
- Fiber: 4g
- Protein: 7g

Lunch

4. Egg Salad Wraps

Preparation Time: 10 minutes

Cooking Time: 0 minutes

Servings: 2

Ingredients:

- 3 tablespoons mayonnaise
- 1 teaspoon Dijon mustard
- 1 tablespoon chopped fresh dill
- ½ teaspoon sea salt
- ¼ teaspoon paprika
- 4 hard-boiled large eggs, chopped
- 1 cup shelled fresh peas
- 2 tablespoons finely chopped red onion
- 2 large kale leaves

Directions:

1. Whisk together the mayonnaise, mustard, dill, salt, and paprika in a medium bowl.
2. Stir in the eggs, peas, and onion.
3. Serve wrapped in kale leaves.

Nutrition:

- Calories: 295 kcal
- Total Fat: 18g
- Saturated Fat: 4g
- Sodium: 620mg
- Carbohydrates: 18g
- Fiber: 4g
- Protein: 17g

5. Pizza Stuffed Pita

Preparation Time: 10 minutes

Cooking Time: 0 minutes

Servings: 2

Ingredients:

- ½ cup tomato sauce
- ½ teaspoon oregano
- ½ teaspoon garlic powder
- ½ cup chopped black olives
- 2 canned artichoke hearts, drained and chopped
- 2 oz. pepperoni, chopped
- ½ cup shredded mozzarella cheese
- 1 whole-wheat pita, halved

Directions:

1. Stir together the tomato sauce, oregano, and garlic powder in a medium bowl.
2. Add the olives, artichoke hearts, pepperoni, and cheese. Stir to mix.
3. Spoon the mixture into the pita halves.

Nutrition:

- Calories: 376 kcal
- Total Fat: 23g
- Saturated Fat: 8g
- Sodium: 1076mg
- Carbohydrates: 27g
- Fiber: 6g
- Protein: 17g

Snack

6. Caprese Skewers

Preparation Time: 5 minutes

Cooking Time: 0 minutes

Servings: 2

Ingredients:

- 12 cherry tomatoes
- 12 basil leaves
- 8 (1-inch) pieces mozzarella cheese
- ¼ cup Italian Vinaigrette (optional, for serving)

Directions:

1. On each of 4 wooden skewers, thread the following: 1 tomato, 1 basil leaf, 1 piece of cheese, 1 tomato, 1 basil leaf, 1 piece of cheese, 1 basil leaf, 1 tomato.
2. Serve with the vinaigrette, if desired, for dipping.

Nutrition:

- Calories: 338 kcal
- Total Fat: 24g
- Saturated Fat: 14g
- Sodium: 672mg
- Carbohydrates: 6g
- Fiber: 1g
- Protein: 25g

Dinner

7. Minestrone

Preparation Time: 10 minutes

Cooking Time: 20 minutes

Servings: 2

Ingredients:

- 1 tablespoon extra-virgin olive oil
- ½ chopped onion
- ½ seeded and chopped red bell pepper
- 1 garlic clove, minced
- 1 cup green bean (fresh or frozen; halved if fresh)
- 3 cups low-sodium vegetable broth
- ½ (14 oz.) can crushed tomatoes
- ½ tablespoon Italian seasoning
- 4 cup dried whole-wheat elbow macaroni
- 4 teaspoon sea salt
- Pinch red pepper flakes (or to taste)

Directions:

1. In a large pot, the olive oil is heated over medium heat until it shimmers. Add the onion and bell pepper and cook, stirring occasionally, until they soften, about 3 minutes. Add the garlic and cook, stirring constantly, for 30 seconds. Add the green beans, vegetable broth, tomatoes, and Italian seasoning and bring to a boil.
2. Add the elbow macaroni, salt, and red pepper flakes. Cook, stirring occasionally, until the macaroni is soft, about 8 minutes.

Nutrition:

- Calories: 200 kcal
- Total Fat: 7g
- Saturated Fat: 1g
- Sodium: 477mg

- Carbohydrates: 29g
- Fiber: 7g
- Protein: 5g

8. Zoodles with Pea Pesto

Preparation Time: 10 minutes

Cooking Time: 10 minutes

Servings: 2

Ingredients:

- 1 ½ zucchini
- 1 tablespoon extra-virgin olive oil
- Pinch sea salt
- Pea Pesto

Directions:

1. Cut the zucchini lengthwise into long strips using a vegetable peeler. Use a knife to cut the strips into the desired width. Alternatively, use a spiralizer to cut the zucchini into noodles.
2. In a large skillet, the olive oil is heated until it shimmers over medium-high heat. Add the zucchini and cook until softened for about 3 minutes. Add the sea salt.
3. Toss the zucchini noodles with the pesto.

Nutrition:

- Calories: 348 kcal
- Total Fat: 30g
- Saturated Fat: 5g
- Sodium: 343mg
- Carbohydrates: 13g
- Fiber: 1g
- Protein: 10g

Chapter 8. Week 2 Meal Plan: Healthy and Omnivorous and Weekly Shopping List

Breakfast

9. Pumpkin Walnut Smoothie Bowl

Preparation Time: 5 minutes

Cooking Time: 0 minutes

Servings: 2

Ingredients:

- 1 cup plain Greek yogurt
- ½ cup canned pumpkin purée (not pumpkin pie mix)
- 1 teaspoon pumpkin pie spice
- 2 (1-gram) packets stevia
- ½ teaspoon vanilla extract
- Pinch sea salt
- ½ cup chopped walnuts

Directions:

1. In a bowl, whisk together the yogurt, pumpkin purée, pumpkin pie spice, stevia, vanilla, and salt (or blend in a blender).
2. Spoon into two bowls. Serve topped with the chopped walnuts.

Nutrition:

- Calories: 292 kcal
- Total Fat: 23g
- Saturated Fat: 4g
- Sodium: 85mg
- Carbohydrates: 15g
- Fiber: 4g
- Protein: 9g

10. Avocado Toast with Tomato and Cottage Cheese

Preparation Time: 5 minutes

Cooking Time: 0 minutes

Servings: 2

Ingredients:

- ½ cup cottage cheese
- ½ avocado, mashed
- 1 teaspoon Dijon mustard
- Dash hot sauce (optional)
- 2 slices whole-grain bread, toasted
- 2 slices tomato

Directions:

1. Mix together the cottage cheese, avocado, mustard, and hot sauce, if using, until well mixed in a small bowl.
2. Spread the mixture on the toast.
3. Top each piece of toast with a tomato slice.

Nutrition:

- Calories: 179 kcal
- Total Fat: 8g
- Saturated Fat: 2g
- Sodium: 327mg
- Carbohydrates: 17g
- Fiber: 4g
- Protein: 11g

Snack

11. Turkey Roll-Ups with Veggie Cream Cheese

Preparation Time: 10 minutes

Cooking Time: 0 minutes

Servings: 2

Ingredients:

- ¼ cup cream cheese, at room temperature
- 2 tablespoons finely chopped red onion
- 2 tablespoons finely chopped red bell pepper
- 1 tablespoon chopped fresh chives
- 1 teaspoon Dijon mustard
- 1 garlic clove, minced
- ¼ teaspoon sea salt
- 6 slices deli turkey

Directions:

1. The cream cheese, red onion, bell pepper, chives, mustard, garlic, and salt are mixed in a small bowl.
2. Spread the mixture on the turkey slices and roll-up.

Nutrition:

- Calories: 146 kcal
- Total Fat: 10g
- Saturated Fat: 6g
- Sodium: 914mg
- Carbohydrates: 5g
- Fiber: 1g
- Protein: 8g

Lunch

12. Almond Butter Apple Pita Pockets

Preparation Time: 10 minutes

Cooking Time: 0 minutes

Servings: 2

Ingredients:

- ½ apple, cored and chopped
- ¼ cup almond butter
- ½ teaspoon cinnamon
- 1 whole-wheat pita, halved

Directions:

1. Stir together the apple, almond butter, and cinnamon in a medium bowl.
2. Spread with a spoon into the pita pocket halves.

Nutrition:

- Calories: 313 kcal
- Total Fat: 20g
- Saturated Fat: 2g
- Sodium: 174mg
- Carbohydrates: 31g
- Fiber: 7g
- Protein: 8g

13. Mason Jar Pear, Walnut, and Spinach Salad

Preparation Time: 10 minutes

Cooking Time: 0 minutes

Servings: 2

Ingredients:

- 4 cups baby spinach
- ½ pear, cored, peeled, and chopped

- ¼ cup whole walnuts, chopped
- 2 tablespoons apple cider vinegar
- 2 tablespoons extra-virgin olive oil
- 1 teaspoon peeled and grated fresh ginger
- ½ teaspoon Dijon mustard
- ½ teaspoon sea salt

Directions:

1. Layer the spinach on the bottom of two mason jars. Top with the pear and walnuts.
2. In a small bowl, whisk together the vinegar, oil, ginger, mustard, and salt. Put in another lidded container.
3. Shake the dressing before serving and add it to the mason jars. Close the jars and shake to distribute the dressing.

Nutrition:

- Calories: 254 kcal
- Total Fat: 23g
- Saturated Fat: 3g
- Sodium: 340mg
- Carbohydrates: 10g
- Fiber: 4g
- Protein: 4g

Snacks

14. Baked Parmesan Crisps

Preparation Time: 5 minutes

Cooking Time: 5 minutes

Servings: 2

Ingredients:

- 1 cup grated Parmesan cheese

Directions:

1. Preheat the oven to 400°F. A rimmed baking sheet is lined with parchment paper.
2. Spread the Parmesan on the prepared baking sheet into 4 mounds, spreading each mound out so it is flat but not touching the others.
3. Bake until brown and crisp, 3 to 5 minutes.
4. Cool for 5 minutes. Use a spatula to remove to a plate to continue cooling.

Nutrition:

- Calories: 216 kcal
- Total Fat: 14g
- Saturated Fat: 9g
- Sodium: 765mg
- Carbohydrates: 2g
- Fiber: 0g
- Protein: 19g

Dinner

15. Shrimp Peri-Peri

Preparation Time: 10 minutes

Cooking Time: 15 minutes

Servings: 2

Ingredients:

- Peri-Peri Sauce
- ½ lb. large shrimp, shelled and deveined
- 1 tablespoon extra-virgin olive oil
- Sea salt

Directions:

1. Preheat the oven broiler on high.
2. In a small pot, bring the Peri-Peri Sauce to a simmer.
3. Meanwhile, place the cleaned shrimp on a rimmed baking sheet, deveined-side down. Brush with olive oil and sprinkle with salt.
4. Broil until opaque, about 5 minutes. Serve with the sauce on the side for dipping or spooned over the top of the shrimp.

Nutrition:

- Calories: 279 kcal
- Total Fat: 16g
- Saturated Fat: 2g
- Sodium: 464mg
- Carbohydrates: 10g
- Fiber: 3g
- Protein: 24g

16. Halibut with Lime and Cilantro

Preparation Time: 30 minutes

Cooking Time: 45 minutes

Servings: 2

Ingredients:

- 2 tablespoons lime juice
- 1 tablespoon chopped fresh cilantro
- 1 teaspoon olive or canola oil
- 1 clove garlic, finely chopped
- 2 halibut or salmon steaks (about ¾ lb.)
- Freshly ground pepper to taste
- ½ cup chunky-style salsa

Directions:

1. In a shallow glass or plastic dish or in a resealable food-storage plastic bag, mix lime juice, cilantro, oil, and garlic. Add halibut, turning several times to coat with marinade. Cover; refrigerate 15 minutes, turning once.
2. Heat gas or charcoal grill. Remove halibut from marinade; discard marinade.
3. Place halibut on the grill over medium heat. Cover grill; cook 10 to 20 minutes, turning once, until halibut flakes easily with a fork. Sprinkle it with pepper. Serve with salsa.

Nutrition:

- Calories: 190 kcal
- Calories from Fat: 40
- Total Fat: 4.5g
- Saturated Fat: 1g
- Trans Fat: 0g
- Cholesterol: 90mg
- Sodium: 600mg
- Total Carbohydrates: 6g
- Dietary Fiber: 0g
- Sugars: 2g
- Protein: 32g

Chapter 9. Week 3 Meal Plan: Healthy and Omnivorous and Weekly Shopping List

Breakfast

17. Nutty Steel-cut Oatmeal with Blueberries

Preparation Time: 5 minutes

Cooking Time: 30 minutes

Servings: 2

Ingredients:

- 1 ½ cups water
- ½ cup steel-cut oats
- 1 ½ tablespoons almond butter
- ½ teaspoon ground cinnamon
- ¼ teaspoon ground nutmeg
- Pinch ground ginger
- ½ cup blueberries
- ¼ cup whole almonds

Directions:

1. Over high-heat, put the water in a medium saucepan, and bring the liquid to a boil.
2. Stir in the oats, and reduce the heat to low so they simmer gently.
3. Simmer the oats uncovered for about 20 minutes, until they are tender.
4. Stir in the almond butter, cinnamon, nutmeg, and ginger, and simmer for an additional 10 minutes.
5. Serve topped with blueberries and whole almonds.

Nutrition:

- Calories: 246 kcal
- Carbohydrates: 24g
- Glycemic Load: 17
- Fiber: 5g
- Protein: 8g
- Sodium: 2mg
- Fat: 14g

18. Quinoa Waffles

Preparation Time: 10 minutes

Cooking Time: 20 minutes

Servings: 2

Ingredients:

- 1 cup unsweetened coconut milk
- ⅛ cup unsweetened applesauce
- 2 eggs
- ⅔ cups quinoa flour
- ¼ cup almond flour
- ½ teaspoon baking powder
- 1 teaspoon ground cinnamon
- Pinch ground ginger
- Pinch sea salt
- 1 tablespoon coconut oil, melted

Directions:

1. Preheat your waffle maker to medium heat.
2. Whisk together the coconut milk, applesauce, and eggs until well blended in a small bowl.
3. In a large bowl, stir together the quinoa flour, almond flour, baking powder, cinnamon, ginger, and salt.
4. Add the wet ingredients to the dry ingredients, and whisk to blend.
5. Brush the waffle iron with coconut oil, and pour ¼ cup of batter into the iron.
6. Cook according to the waffle iron instructions.
7. Repeat with the remaining batter. Serve 2 waffles per person.

Nutrition:

- Calories: 296 kcal
- Carbohydrates: 15g
- Glycemic Load: 19
- Fiber: 1g
- Protein: 20g
- Sodium: 296mg
- Fat: 15g

Snack

19. Garlicky Hummus

Preparation Time: 5 minutes

Cooking Time: 10 minutes

Servings: 2

Ingredients:

- 1½ cups canned chickpeas, rinsed and drained
- ¼ cup tahini
- 2 teaspoons minced garlic
- 1 teaspoon ground cumin
- ½ teaspoon ground coriander
- ¼ cup freshly squeezed lemon juice
- 2 tablespoons olive oil
- Sea salt

Directions:

1. Put the chickpeas, tahini, garlic, cumin, coriander, and lemon juice in a food processor, and blend until smooth, scraping down the sides of the processor at least once.
2. Incorporate the olive oil and process until blended. Season with sea salt.
3. Store the hummus in a sealed container in the refrigerator for up to 1 week.

Nutrition:

- Calories: 147 kcal
- Carbohydrates: 14g
- Glycemic Load: 10
- Fiber: 4g
- Protein: 5g
- Sodium: 35mg
- Fat: 9g

Lunch

20. Mediterranean Steak Sandwiches

Preparation Time: 1 hour

Cooking Time: 10 minutes

Servings: 2

Ingredients:

- 1 tablespoon extra-virgin olive oil
- 1 tablespoon balsamic vinegar
- 1 teaspoon garlic
- 1 teaspoon lemon juice
- 1 teaspoon fresh oregano
- ½ teaspoon fresh parsley
- ½-pound flank steak
- 2 whole-wheat pitas
- 1 cup shredded lettuce
- ½ red onion, thinly sliced
- ½ tomato, chopped
- ½ oz. low-sodium feta cheese

Directions:

1. Scourge olive oil, balsamic vinegar, garlic, lemon juice, oregano, and parsley.
2. Add the steak to the bowl, turning to coat it completely.
3. Marinate the steak for 1 hour in the refrigerator, turning it over several times.
4. Preheat the broiler. Line a baking sheet with aluminum foil.
5. Put steak out of the bowl and discard the marinade.
6. Situate steak on the baking sheet and broil for 5 minutes per side for medium.
7. Set aside for 10 minutes before slicing.
8. Stuff the pitas with the sliced steak, lettuce, onion, tomato, and feta.

Nutrition:

- Calories: 344 kcal
- Carbohydrates: 22g
- Fiber: 3g

21. Chicken and Roasted Vegetable Wraps

Preparation Time: 10 minutes

Cooking Time: 20 minutes

Servings: 2

Ingredients:

- ¼ small eggplant
- ½ red bell pepper
- ½ medium zucchini
- ¼ small red onion, sliced
- ½ tablespoon extra-virgin olive oil
- 1 (8 oz.) cooked chicken breasts, sliced
- 2 whole-wheat tortilla wraps

Directions:

1. Preheat the oven to 400°F.
2. Wrap the baking sheet with foil and set it aside.
3. In a large bowl, toss the eggplant, bell pepper, zucchini, and red onion with the olive oil.
4. Transfer the vegetables to the baking sheet and lightly season with salt and pepper.
5. Roast the vegetables until soft and slightly charred, about 20 minutes.
6. Divide the vegetables and chicken into four portions.
7. Wrap 1 tortilla around each portion of chicken and grilled vegetables, and serve.

Nutrition:

- Calories: 483
- Carbohydrates: 45g
- Fiber: 3g

Snack

22. Pesto Veggie Pizza

Preparation Time: 20 minutes

Cooking Time: 15 minutes

Servings: 2

Ingredients:

- Olive oil, for greasing the parchment paper
- ¼ head cauliflower, cut into florets
- 3 tablespoons almond flour
- ½ teaspoons olive oil
- 1 egg, beaten
- Minced garlic
- Pinch sea salt
- ¼ cup Simple Tomato Sauce (here)
- ¼ zucchini, thinly sliced
- ¼ cup baby spinach leaves
- 2 ½ asparagus spears, woody ends trimmed, cut into 3-inch pieces
- Basil pesto

Directions:

1. Preheat the oven to 450°F. Put a baking sheet without a rim in the oven.
2. Prepare a piece of parchment paper by lightly brushing with olive oil, and set aside.
3. Put a large saucepan filled halfway with water over high heat, and bring it to a boil.
4. Put the cauliflower in a food processor, and pulse until very finely chopped, almost flour consistency.
5. Transfer the ground cauliflower to a fine-mesh sieve, and put it over the boiling water for about 1 minute, until the cauliflower is cooked.
6. Wring out all the water from the cauliflower using a kitchen towel. Transfer the cauliflower to a large bowl.

7. Stir in the almond flour, oil, egg, garlic, and salt, and mix to create a thick dough. Use your hands to press the ingredients together, and transfer the cauliflower mixture to the parchment paper.
8. Press the mixture out into a flat circle, about ½ inch thick. Slide the parchment paper onto the baking sheet in the oven.
9. Bake the crust for about 10 minutes, until it is crisp and turns golden brown.
10. Remove the crust from the oven, and spread the sauce evenly to the edges of the crust.
11. Arrange the zucchini, spinach, and asparagus on the pizza.
12. Drizzle the pizza with basil pesto, and put it back in the oven for about 2 minutes, until the vegetables are tender. Serve.

Nutrition:

- Calories: 107 kcal
- Carbohydrates: 8g
- Glycemic Load: 5
- Fiber: 3g
- Protein: 5g
- Sodium: 64mg
- Fat: 7g

Dinner

23. Pork Chop Diane

Preparation Time: 10 minutes

Cooking Time: 20 minutes

Servings: 2

Ingredients:

- 8 cup low-sodium chicken broth
- ½ tablespoon freshly squeezed lemon juice
- 1 teaspoon Worcestershire sauce
- 1 teaspoon Dijon mustard
- 2 (5 oz.) boneless pork top loin chops
- ½ teaspoon extra-virgin olive oil
- ½ teaspoon lemon zest
- ½ teaspoon butter
- 1 teaspoon chopped fresh chives

Directions:

1. Blend together the chicken broth, lemon juice, Worcestershire sauce, and Dijon mustard and set it aside.
2. Season the pork chops lightly.
3. Situate a large skillet over medium-high heat and add the olive oil.
4. Cook the pork chops, turning once, until they are no longer pink, about 8 minutes per side.
5. Put aside the chops.
6. Pour the broth mixture into the skillet and cook until warmed through and thickened, about 2 minutes.
7. Blend lemon zest, butter, and chives.
8. Garnish with a generous spoonful of sauce.

Nutrition:

- Calories: 200 kcal
- Fat: 8g
- Carbohydrates: 1g

24. Autumn Pork Chops with Red Cabbage and Apples

Preparation Time: 15 minutes

Cooking Time: 30 minutes

Servings: 2

Ingredients:

- ⅛ cup apple cider vinegar
- 1 tablespoon granulated sweetener
- 2 (4 oz.) pork chops, about 1 inch thick
- ½ tablespoon extra-virgin olive oil
- ¼ red cabbage, finely shredded
- ½ sweet onion, thinly sliced
- ½ apple, peeled, cored, and sliced
- ½ teaspoon chopped fresh thyme

Directions:

1. Scourge together the vinegar and sweetener. Set it aside.
2. Season the pork with salt and pepper.
3. Position a big skillet over medium-high heat and add the olive oil.
4. Cook the pork chops until no longer pink, turning once, about 8 minutes per side.
5. Put chops aside.
6. Add the cabbage and onion to the skillet and sauté until the vegetables have softened about 5 minutes.
7. Add the vinegar mixture and the apple slices to the skillet and bring the mixture to boiling point.
8. Adjust low-heat and simmer for 5 additional minutes.
9. Return the pork chops to the skillet, along with any accumulated juices and thyme, cover, and cook for 5 more minutes.

Nutrition:

- Calories: 223 kcal
- Fat: 12g
- Carbohydrates: 3g

Chapter 10. Week 4 Meal Plan: Healthy and Omnivorous and Weekly Shopping List

Breakfast

25. Toasty Oatmeal Pancakes

Preparation Time: 10 minutes

Cooking Time: 21 minutes

Servings: 2

Ingredients:

- 1 cup rolled oats
- 1 cup unsweetened almond milk
- ¼ cup almond flour
- ½ teaspoon baking soda
- ½ teaspoon baking powder
- ¼ teaspoon ground cinnamon
- ¼ teaspoon ground nutmeg
- Pinch sea salt
- 1 egg, at room temperature, beaten
- ⅛ cup melted coconut oil, plus extra for cooking
- ½ teaspoon pure vanilla extract

Directions:

1. Mix the oats and almond milk in a large bowl, and set aside for at least 2 hours (up to overnight) to soften the oats.
2. When you are ready to make the pancakes, in a small bowl, stir together the almond flour, baking soda, baking powder, cinnamon, nutmeg, and salt.
3. Whisk the eggs, melted oil, and vanilla into the oat mixture until blended.

4. Combine the dry ingredients by stirring them into the wet ingredients until just mixed.
5. Put a large skillet over medium heat, and brush the skillet with oil.
6. Pour the batter into the skillet, ¼ cup per pancake, and cook for about 4 minutes, until the edges are firm and the bottoms golden.
7. The pancakes are flipped and cooked until the second side is golden and the pancake is cooked through for about 3 minutes.
8. Repeat with the remaining batter. Serve 3 pancakes per person.

Nutrition:

- Calories: 353 kcal
- Carbohydrates: 31g
- Glycemic Load: 15
- Fiber: 5g
- Protein: 9g
- Sodium: 499mg
- Fat: 23g

26. Tomato-Herb Omelet

Preparation Time: 10 minutes

Cooking Time: 10 minutes

Servings: 2

Ingredients:

- 1 tablespoon coconut oil, divided
- 2 scallions, green and white parts, chopped
- 1 teaspoon minced garlic
- 2 tomatoes, chopped, liquid squeezed out
- 6 eggs, beaten
- ½ teaspoon chopped fresh thyme
- ½ teaspoon chopped fresh basil
- ½ teaspoon chopped fresh chives
- ½ teaspoon chopped fresh oregano
- ⅛ teaspoon sea salt
- Pinch ground nutmeg
- Pinch freshly ground black pepper
- Chopped fresh parsley, for garnish

Directions:

1. Put a small saucepan over medium heat before adding 1 teaspoon of coconut oil.
2. Sauté the scallions and garlic for about 3 minutes, until the vegetables are softened.
3. Add the tomatoes and sauté for 3 minutes. Remove the saucepan from the heat and set aside.
4. Whisk together the eggs, thyme, basil, chives, oregano, salt, nutmeg, and pepper in a medium bowl.
5. Put a large skillet over medium-high heat before adding the remaining 2 teaspoons of oil. Swirl the oil until it coats the skillet.
6. Pour in the egg mixture, and swirl until the eggs start to firm up—do not stir the eggs. Lift the edges of the firmed eggs to let the uncooked egg flow at the bottom.
7. When the eggs are almost done, spoon the tomato mixture onto one-half of the eggs.

8. Fold the uncovered side over the tomato mixture and cook for a minute longer.
9. Cut the omelet in half, sprinkle with parsley, and serve.

Nutrition:

- Calories: 306 kcal
- Carbohydrates: 13g
- Glycemic Load: 3
- Fiber: 6g
- Protein: 19g
- Sodium: 312mg
- Fat: 21g

Snack

27. Apple Leather

Preparation Time: 10 minutes

Cooking Time: 8 to 10 hours

Servings: 24 strips

Ingredients:

- 5 apples, peeled, cored, and sliced
- ¼ cup water
- 1 teaspoon pure vanilla extract
- ¼ teaspoon ground ginger
- ¼ teaspoon ground cloves

Directions:

1. Put the apples, water, vanilla, ginger, and cloves in a large saucepan over medium heat.
2. Bring the mixture to a boil, reduce to low heat, and simmer for about 20 minutes, until the apples are very tender.
3. Transfer the apple mixture to a food processor, and purée until very smooth.
4. Set the oven on the lowest possible setting.
5. Line a baking sheet with parchment paper.
6. Pour the puréed apple mixture onto the baking sheet, and spread it out very thinly and evenly.
7. Place the baking sheet in the oven, and bake for 8 to 10 hours, until the leather is smooth and no longer sticky.
8. Cut the apple leather with a pizza cutter into 24 strips, and store this treat in a sealed container in a cool, dark place for up to 2 weeks.

Nutrition:

- Calories: 41 kcal
- Carbohydrates: 11g
- Glycemic Load: 2

- Fiber: 2g
- Protein: 0g
- Sodium: 1mg
- Fat: 0g

Lunch

28. Almond-Crusted Salmon

Preparation Time: 10 minutes

Cooking Time: 15 minutes

Servings: 2

Ingredients:

- ⅛ cup almond meal
- ⅛ cup whole-wheat breadcrumbs
- ⅛ teaspoon ground coriander
- 1/16 teaspoon ground cumin
- 2 (6 oz.) boneless salmon fillets
- ½ tablespoon fresh lemon juice
- Salt and pepper

Directions:

1. Ready the oven at 500°F and line a small baking dish with foil.
2. Combine the almond meal, breadcrumbs, coriander, and cumin in a small bowl.
3. Rinse the fish in cool water then pat dry and brush with lemon juice.
4. Season the fish with salt and pepper then dredge in the almond mixture on both sides.
5. Situate fish in the baking dish and bake for 15 minutes.

Nutrition:

- Calories: 232 kcal
- Carbohydrates: 5.8g
- Sugar: 1.7g

29. Chicken & Veggie Bowl with Brown Rice

Preparation Time: 10 minutes

Cooking Time: 20 minutes

Servings: 2

Ingredients:

- ½ cup instant brown rice
- ⅛ cup tahini
- ⅛ cup fresh lemon juice
- 1 clove minced garlic
- ⅛ teaspoon ground cumin
- Pinch salt
- ½ tablespoon olive oil
- 2 (4 oz.) chicken breast halves
- ¼ medium yellow onion, sliced
- 1 cup green beans, trimmed
- 1 cup chopped broccoli
- 2 cups chopped kale

Directions:

1. Bring 1-cup of water to boil in a small saucepan.
2. Stir in the brown rice and simmer for 5 minutes then cover and set aside.
3. Meanwhile, whisk together the tahini with ¼-cup water in a small bowl.
4. Stir in the lemon juice, garlic, and cumin with a pinch of salt and stir well.
5. Heat up oil in a big cast-iron skillet over medium heat.
6. Season the chicken with salt and pepper then add to the skillet.
7. Cook for 3 to 5 minutes on each side until cooked through then remove to a cutting board and cover loosely with foil.
8. Reheat the skillet and cook the onion for 2 minutes then stir in the broccoli and beans.
9. Sauté for 2 minutes then stir in the kale and sauté 2 minutes more.
10. Add 2 tablespoons of water then cover and steam for 2 minutes while you slice the chicken.

11. Build the bowls with brown rice, sliced chicken, and sautéed veggies.
12. Serve hot drizzled with the lemon tahini dressing.

Nutrition:

- Calories: 435 kcal
- Carbohydrates: 24g
- Sugar: 4.8g

Snack

30. Simple Appetizer Meatballs

Preparation Time: 25 minutes

Cooking Time: 25 minutes

Servings: 24 pieces

Ingredients:

- ½ pound lean ground beef
- ½ pound lean ground pork
- ½ cup sodium-free chicken broth
- ¼ cup almond flour
- 1 tablespoon low-sodium tamari sauce
- ½ teaspoon ground cumin
- ¼ teaspoon freshly ground black pepper

Directions:

1. Preheat the oven to 375°F.
2. Combine all the ingredients together until completely incorporated in a large bowl.
3. Roll the mixture into ¾-inch balls, and place them on a parchment-lined baking sheet.
4. Bake the meatballs for 25 to 30 minutes, until they are cooked through and golden brown.
5. Serve.

Nutrition:

- Calories: 125 kcal
- Carbohydrates: 0g
- Glycemic Load: 0
- Fiber: 0g
- Protein: 20g
- Sodium: 157mg
- Fat: 4g

Dinner

31. Chipotle Chili Pork Chops

Preparation Time: 4 hours

Cooking Time: 20 minutes

Servings: 2

Ingredients:

- Juice and zest of ½ lime
- ½ tablespoon extra-virgin olive oil
- ½ tablespoon chipotle chili powder
- 1 teaspoon minced garlic
- ½ teaspoon ground cinnamon
- Pinch sea salt
- 2 (5 oz.) pork chops

Directions:

1. Combine the lime juice and zest, oil, chipotle chili powder, garlic, cinnamon, and salt in a resealable plastic bag. Add the pork chops. Remove as much air as possible and seal the bag.
2. Marinate the chops in the refrigerator for at least 4 hours, and up to 24 hours, turning them several times.
3. Ready the oven to 400°F and set a rack on a baking sheet. Let the chops rest at room temperature for 15 minutes, then arrange them on the rack and discard the remaining marinade.
4. Roast the chops until cooked through, turning once, about 10 minutes per side.
5. Serve with lime wedges.

Nutrition:

- Calories: 205 kcal
- Carbohydrates: 1g
- Sugar: 1g

32. Orange-Marinated Pork Tenderloin

Preparation Time: 2 hours

Cooking Time: 30 minutes

Servings: 2

Ingredients:

- ⅛ cup freshly squeezed orange juice
- 1 teaspoon orange zest
- 1 teaspoon minced garlic
- ½ teaspoon low-sodium soy sauce
- ½ teaspoon grated fresh ginger
- ½ teaspoon honey
- ¾ pounds pork tenderloin roast
- ½ tablespoon extra-virgin olive oil

Directions:

1. Blend together the orange juice, zest, garlic, soy sauce, ginger, and honey.
2. Pour the marinade into a resealable plastic bag and add the pork tenderloin.
3. Remove as much air as possible and seal the bag. Marinate the pork in the refrigerator, turning the bag a few times, for 2 hours.
4. Preheat the oven to 400°F.
5. Pull out tenderloin from the marinade and discard the marinade.
6. Position a big ovenproof skillet over medium-high heat and add the oil.
7. Sear the pork tenderloin on all sides, about 5 minutes in total.
8. Position skillet to the oven and roast for 25 minutes.
9. Put aside for 10 minutes before serving.

Nutrition:

- Calories: 228 kcal
- Carbohydrates: 4g
- Sugar: 3g

Chapter 11. Week 1 Meal Plan: Vegetarian and Weekly Shopping List

Breakfast

33. Broccoli Omelet

Preparation Time: 5 minutes

Cooking Time: 1.5-2 hours

Servings: 2

Ingredients:

- 2 garlic cloves, minced
- 3 eggs
- ½ yellow onion, chopped
- ¼ cup milk
- ½ cup broccoli florets, fresh or frozen
- ¼ teaspoon black pepper
- ½ tomato, chopped
- ⅛ teaspoon chili powder
- ½ tablespoon Parmesan cheese, shredded
- ¾ cups Cheddar cheese, shredded
- ⅛ teaspoon salt
- ⅛ cup green onions, chopped
- ⅛ teaspoon garlic powder

Directions:

1. Whisk the eggs, milk, and spices in a bowl.
2. To the egg mixture, add onions along with the garlic, parmesan cheese, and broccoli. Stir well until combined, and then pour the egg mixture into a slow cooker.
3. Close the lid and cook for about 1 ½ hour to 2 hours on high.

4. Remove the cover when the cooking time is over and then sprinkle the shredded cheddar cheese on top. Close the lid again and then turn off the slow cooker.
5. Let rest for about 10 minutes, until the cheddar cheese has melted.
6. When done, cut the omelet into quarters and then serve.
7. Garnish the servings with chopped green onion and fresh tomato. Enjoy!

Nutrition:

- Calories: 423 kcal
- Fat: 28g
- Carbohydrates: 13g
- Protein: 29g

34. Wild Rice

Preparation Time: 5 minutes

Cooking Time: 2-3 hours

Servings: 2

Ingredients:

- ¼ cup onions, diced
- ½ cup wild rice, or wild rice mixture, uncooked
- ¾ cups chicken broth, low sodium
- ¼ cup diced green or red peppers
- ⅛ teaspoon pepper
- ½ tablespoon oil
- ⅛ teaspoon salt
- ¼ cup mushrooms, sliced

Directions:

1. In a slow cooker, layer the rice and the vegetables, and then pour oil, pepper, and salt over the vegetables. Stir well.
2. Heat the chicken broth in a pot, and then pour over the ingredients in the slow cooker.
3. Close the lid and cook for 2 ½-3 hours on high, until the rice has softened and the liquid is absorbed.
4. Serve and enjoy!

Nutrition:

- Calories: 157 kcal
- Fat: 3g
- Carbohydrates: 27g
- Protein: 6g

Snack

35. French Bread Pizza

Preparation Time: 5 minutes

Cooking Time: 2-3 hours

Servings: 2

Ingredients:

- ½ cup asparagus(diced)
- ½ cup Roma tomatoes(diced)
- ½ cup red bell pepper(diced)
- ½ tablespoon minced garlic
- ½ loaf French bread
- ½ cup pizza sauce
- ½ cup low-fat shredded mozzarella cheese

Directions:

1. Heat the oven to 400°F. Coat the baking sheet lightly with a cooking spray.
2. Add the asparagus, tomatoes, and pepper in a little dish. Add the garlic and stir gently to coat uniformly.
3. Adjust the French bread to the baking sheet. Apply ¼ cup of the pizza sauce and ¼ of the vegetable paste to each portion of the mixture. Sprinkle with ¼ cup of mozzarella cheese.
4. Bake until the cheese is finely browned and the vegetables are tender for 8 to 10 minutes. Serve straight away.

Nutrition:

- Calories: 265 kcal
- Total Fat: 5g
- Saturated Fat: 2g
- Trans Fat: 0g
- Total Carbohydrates: 40g
- Dietary Fiber: 4g
- Added Sugars: 0g
- Protein: 15g

Lunch

36. Spinach Lasagna

Preparation Time: 5 minutes

Cooking Time: 2-3 hours

Servings: 2

Ingredients:

- Parmesan cheese, freshly grated
- 3 lasagna noodles, gluten-free or whole-wheat
- 1 oz. tomato sauce, unsalted
- 4 ½ oz. jarred pasta tomato sauce, lower sodium
- 1 cooking spray, nonstick
- Mozzarella cheese, part-skim, shredded, divided
- Ricotta cheese, low-fat
- 10 oz. spinach, frozen, chopped, thawed, drained

Directions:

1. Generously spray a Crockpot with a nonstick cooking spray.
2. Mix ricotta cheese together with ¼ cup of mozzarella cheese, spinach, and parmesan cheese in a bowl.
3. Evenly spread a cup of pasta sauce at the bottom of the crockpot, and then side by side arrange 3 noodles on top of the spread sauce, as you break the noodles.
4. On top of the noodles, spread about ⅓ cup of the ricotta-spinach mixture, and then repeat the layering with the pasta sauce, noodles, and then the ricotta-spinach mixture, 2 more times. Finally, top with the rest of the pasta sauce and the canned tomato sauce, and then sprinkle 1 cup of the mozzarella cheese on top.
5. When done, close the lid and cook for about 2-3 hours on low. Serve and enjoy!

Nutrition:

- Calories: 180 kcal
- Fat: 6g

- Total Carbohydrates: 22g
- Protein: 10g

37. Mushroom Soup with Sherry

Preparation Time: 5 minutes

Cooking Time: 5 hours

Servings: 2

Ingredients:

- 1 teaspoon cassava flour
- ⅔ cups boiling water
- ⅓ cups dried porcini mushrooms
- ⅙ tablespoon soy sauce
- ⅓ tablespoons olive oil
- Garlic clove, minced
- ⅓ cups shallots, sliced
- ⅓ cup dry sherry
- Heavy cream
- Thyme, chopped
- ½ lb. assorted fresh mushrooms, sliced
- A pinch of salt
- A pinch of black pepper

Directions:

1. Pour 2 cups boiling water over the porcini mushrooms. Let rest for 20 minutes. Drain the porcini mushrooms in a colander over a bowl and reserve the mushroom broth. Set mushrooms aside.
2. Strain mushroom broth into a bowl. Remove solids. Add soy sauce, cassava flour, salt, pepper, and remaining boiling water into the broth and set aside.
3. Over medium heat, heat oil in a skillet. Add garlic and shallots and let it cook for 5 minutes. Add sherry, bring to boil, and cook for 30 seconds. Remove from heat.
4. Add the broth mixture, porcini mushrooms, shallot mixture, fresh mushrooms, and thyme to a slow cooker. Cover and cook for 4 hours on high heat. Uncover and cook for 20 minutes. Transfer 2 cups of soup to a blender. Cover the lid. Blend for 10 seconds.
5. Add the pureed soup to the cooker. Add the cream. Transfer to bowls. Serve.

Nutrition:

- Calories: 101 kcal
- Fat: 5g
- Total Carbohydrates: 11g
- Protein: 5g

Snack

38. Spicy Bruschetta

Preparation Time: 5 minutes

Cooking Time: 10 minutes

Servings: 2

Ingredients:

- 1 baguette roll
- Salt and white pepper
- ½ tomato
- ½ tbsp. acetic balsamic vinegar
- 37.5 g roasted peppers from the jar
- 2 tbsps. oil
- ½ clove of garlic
- 1 red chili
- ½ onion

Directions:

1. Halve the rolls and drizzle with 1 tablespoon of oil.
2. Preheat the oven to 200°C and roast the rolls on both sides for 2-3 minutes.
3. Pour boiling water over the tomato and let it steep for a moment. Then peel and core the tomato and dice the pulp.
4. Drain the peppers and cut them into small pieces. Peel and dice the garlic. Peel and chop the onion. Core the chili pepper and cut it into slices.
5. Mix all ingredients with 3 tablespoons of oil and vinegar. Season the mixture with salt and pepper.
6. Spread the vegetables on the rolls and briefly heat them again in the oven.

Nutrition:

- Calories: 205 kcal
- Fat: 10.4g

- Carbohydrates: 23.6g
- Protein: 3.8g

Dinner

39. Vegetarian Chipotle Chili

Preparation Time: 5 minutes

Cooking Time: 6 hours

Servings: 2

Ingredients:

- ¼ onion, diced
- 2 ¼ oz. corn, frozen
- ¾ carrots, diced
- Ground cumin
- 1 garlic clove, minced
- ½ medium sweet potatoes, diced
- ¼ teaspoon chipotle chili powder
- Ground black pepper
- 1 cup kidney beans, cooked from dried beans, or use rinsed canned beans
- ¼ tablespoon salt
- 7 oz. tomatoes, diced, undrained
- ½ avocados, diced

Directions:

1. In a slow cooker, combine all the ingredients except the diced avocados.
2. Cook for 3 hours on high, and then cook for 3 hours on low until done. If desired, you can also cook for 4-5 hours on high or 7-8 hours on low until cooked through.
3. When done, serve with the diced avocado and enjoy!

Nutrition:

- Calories: 283 kcal
- Fat: 8g
- Carbohydrates: 45g
- Protein: 11g

40. Crock Pot Veggies Soup

Preparation Time: 5 minutes

Cooking Time: 4-6 hours

Servings: 2

Ingredients:

- 1 garlic clove, minced
- 4 ⅔ oz. tomatoes, diced, with juice
- 1 celery stalks, diced
- 2 cups vegetable broth, low-sodium
- ⅓ large onion, diced
- 1 cup cabbage, chopped
- 1 large carrot, diced
- ⅓ teaspoon Spike seasoning, salt-free
- ⅓ large sweet potato, peeled & diced
- Salt, optional
- ⅓ medium parsnip, diced
- Black pepper
- ⅓ red bell pepper, seeded & diced

Directions:

1. In a crockpot, stir all the ingredients together, and then set the pot on high.
2. Allow cooking for about 4-6 hours.
3. When through, stir gently and then mash parsnips and sweet potatoes lightly in order to slightly thicken the soup.
4. Serve and enjoy!

Nutrition:

- Calories: 135 kcal
- Fat: 0.5g
- Carbohydrates: 30g
- Protein: 4g

-

Chapter 12. Week 2 Meal Plan: Vegetarian and Weekly Shopping List

Breakfast

41. Butternut Squash Risotto

Preparation Time: 5 minutes

Cooking Time: 1 hour 30 minutes

Servings: 2

Ingredients:

- ½ tablespoon olive oil
- ½ cup Arborio rice
- ¼ cup onion, chopped
- ⅛ teaspoon salt
- 1 ¼ cups vegetable broth, low sodium
- 1 garlic clove, minced
- ¼ teaspoon ground cinnamon
- ⅛ teaspoon pepper
- 1 cup butternut squash, cubed

Directions:

1. Over medium heat, pour oil into a skillet and let it be heated before adding onion along with the garlic. Cook for 3-5 minutes until translucent, and then add rice and allow to heat as you stir occasionally for 3 minutes.
2. When done, add the mixture to a slow cooker, and then add squash along with the broth, cinnamon, salt, and pepper.
3. Close the cover and cook for 1 hour 30 minutes on high until the rice has become tender.
4. Serve and enjoy!

Nutrition:

- Calories: 739 kcal
- Fat: 45.9g
- Carbohydrates: 15g
- Protein: 5g

42. Slow "Roasted" Tomatoes

Preparation Time: 5 minutes

Cooking Time: 1 hour 15 minutes

Servings: 2

Ingredients:

- ½ tablespoon balsamic vinegar
- 1 large firm under-ripe tomato, halved crosswise
- 1 garlic clove, minced
- 1 teaspoon olive oil
- ½ teaspoon dried basil, crushed
- ½ cup breadcrumbs, coarse, soft whole-wheat
- Dried rosemary, crushed
- 1 tablespoon Parmesan cheese, grated
- Salt
- ¼ teaspoon dried oregano, crushed
- Chopped fresh basil, optional

Directions:

1. Using cooking spray, coat the unheated slow cooker lightly. Then add tomatoes to the bottom of the slow cooker, cut side up.
2. In a bowl, combine vinegar together with garlic, oil, rosemary, dried basil, and salt, and then spoon the mixture over the tomatoes in the slow cooker evenly.
3. Close the lid and cook for either 2 hours on low, or 1 hour on high.
4. Over medium heat, preheat a skillet, and then add the breadcrumbs. Cook as you stir constantly until lightly browned, for about 2-3 minutes. Remove from heat when done and then stir in the parmesan.
5. When through, remove tomatoes from the slow cooker and put them on the serving plates, and then drizzle over tomatoes with the cooking liquid. Then sprinkle with the breadcrumb mixture and let rest for 10 minutes in order to absorb the flavors.
6. Garnish with basil if need be and then serve. Enjoy!

Nutrition:

- Calories: 96 kcal

- Fat: 4g
- Carbohydrates: 13g
- Protein: 3g

Snack

43. Easy pizza for two

Preparation Time: 5 minutes

Cooking Time: 10 minutes

Servings: 2

Ingredients:

- ½ cup chunky no-salt-added
- Tomato sauce
- 1 ready-made whole-wheat flatbread (about 10-inch diameter)
- 2 slices of onion, (¼-inch wide)
- 4 sliced red bell pepper (¼-inch wide)
- ½ cup shredded low-fat mozzarella
- 2 tablespoons chopped fresh basil

Directions:

1. Heat the oven to 350°F.
2. Coat the baking pan lightly with the cooking oil.
3. Spread the tomato sauce on the flatbread. Cover with tomato, chili pepper, mozzarella, and basil.
4. Place the pizza in a baking pan and cook until the cheese melts and becomes lightly browned approximately five minutes.

Nutrition:

- Protein: 8g
- Calories: 163 kcal
- Total Fat: 5g
- Total Carbohydrates: 26g
- Dietary Fiber: 6g
- Total Sugars: 8g
- Added Sugars: 0g

Lunch

44. Winter Vegetable Medley

Preparation Time: 5 minutes

Cooking Time: 4-6 hours

Servings: 2

Ingredients:

- ½ teaspoon thyme
- 1 ¼ cups baby carrots
- ½ onion, sliced
- 1 ¼ cups butternut or acorn squash, peeled, chopped
- ¼ teaspoon sea salt
- 1 ¼ cups vegetable broth
- Chopped chives or parsley, to garnish (optional)

Directions:

1. Combine all the ingredients to a slow cooker except chives and parsley.
2. Close the lid and cook for 4-6 hours on low, until the vegetables have become tender.
3. When cooked through, garnish with parsley or chives on top if desired, and then serve topped with chives or parsley. Enjoy!

Nutrition:

- Calories: 128 kcal
- Total Fat: 1g
- Total Carbohydrates: 28g
- Protein: 4g

45. Classic Split Pea Soup

Preparation Time: 5 minutes

Cooking Time: 6-8 hours

Servings: 2

Ingredients:

- ½ cup celery, chopped
- 8 oz. split peas, dried
- 1 ½ cups water
- 1 carrot, chopped
- ¼ teaspoon salt
- ½ cup onion, chopped
- ¼ teaspoon pepper
- ½ cup ham, low-sodium, diced, cooked
- ½ bay leaf
- 2 cups chicken broth, low sodium

Directions:

1. To a slow cooker, add peas along with the remaining ingredients.
2. Close the lid and allow to cook for 8 hours on low until the peas have become tender and the soup has thickened.
3. When through, remove the bay leaf and discard it.
4. Ladle the pea soup to the bowls and then serve immediately. Enjoy!

Nutrition:

- Calories: 243 kcal
- Fat: 14g
- Carbohydrates: 20g
- Protein: 12g

Snack

46. Bean Salad with Balsamic Vinaigrette

Preparation Time: 5 minutes

Cooking Time: 0 hours

Servings: 2

Ingredients:

For the Vinaigrette:

- 2 tablespoons balsamic vinegar
- ⅓ cup fresh parsley, chopped
- 4 garlic cloves, finely chopped
- Ground black pepper, to taste
- ¼ cup Extra-virgin olive oil

For the Salad:

- ⅓ can (15 oz.) low-sodium garbanzo beans, rinsed and drained
- ⅓ can (15 oz.) low-sodium black beans, rinsed and drained
- 1 small red onion, diced
- 2 lettuce leaves
- Celery, finely chopped

Directions:

1. In a small pan, mix the balsamic vinegar, the parsley, the garlic, and the pepper to prepare the vinaigrette. Slowly add the olive oil when whisking.
2. In a large pan, combine the beans and the onion.
3. Pour the vinaigrette over the mixture and stir softly, blend thoroughly and coat equally. Cover and refrigerate until ready to serve.
4. Put one lettuce leaf on each plate to serve. Divide the salad between the individual plates and garnish with the minced celery. Serve straight away.

Nutrition:

- Calories: 206 kcal
- Saturated Fat: 1g
- Total Fat: 10g
- Monounsaturated Fat: 7g
- Total Carbohydrates: 22g
- Dietary Fiber: 8g
- Sodium: 174mg
- Cholesterol: 0mg
- Protein: 7g

Dinner

47. Squash Soup

Preparation Time: 5 minutes

Cooking Time: 4 hours 10 minutes

Servings: 2

Ingredients:

- 1 garlic clove, minced
- 1 sprigs thyme
- 1 small onion, chopped
- 1 small butternut squash, peeled, cut into large cubes
- 1 small carrot, peeled, chopped
- ⅓ sprig sage
- Kosher salt & freshly ground pepper, to taste
- 1 cup chicken or vegetable broth, low sodium
- Cayenne, a pinch
- Freshly chopped parsley, to garnish
- Heavy cream, to serve

Directions:

1. Combine the butternut squash together with carrot, garlic, onion, sage, and thyme in a slow cooker. Then pour in the broth along with salt, cayenne, and pepper to season.
2. Close the lid and cook for 8 hours on low or 4 hours on high, until the squash has become very tender.
3. When through, remove the herbs sprigs and transfer the soup into a blender. Blend the soup until smooth.
4. Stir in the heavy cream and then garnish with chopped parsley.
5. Serve and enjoy!

Nutrition:

- Calories: 243 kcal
- Fat: 14g
- Total Carbohydrates: 20g
- Protein: 12g

48. Easy Nacho Skillet Dinner

Preparation Time: 5 minutes

Cooking Time: 15 minutes

Servings: 2

Ingredients:

- ⅔ cups ground soy crumbles
- ⅔ cups frozen corn
- ⅔ teaspoons chili powder
- ⅓ can (15 oz.) no-salt-added kidney beans, drained and rinsed
- ⅔ cans (8 oz.) no-salt-added tomato sauce
- ⅓ cup water
- ⅓ cup slightly broken baked tortilla chips (about ⅓ oz.)
- Reduced-fat shredded cheddar cheese

Directions:

1. Put meatless ground crumbs, corn, chili powder, kidney beans, tomato sauce, and water in a 10-inch skillet over medium-high heat.
2. Simmer for ten minutes, stirring periodically.
3. Sprinkle with tortilla chips and some cheese. Put the cover and let stand for about 5 minutes before the cheese is melted.

Nutrition:

- Calories: 295 kcal
- Saturated Fat: 2.5g
- Total Fat: 7g
- Trans Fat: 0g
- Total Carbohydrates: 39g
- Dietary Fiber: 12g
- Added Sugars: 0g
- Protein: 19g

Chapter 13. Week 3 Meal Plan: Vegetarian and Weekly Shopping List

Breakfast

49. Coconut and Berry Smoothie

Preparation Time: 5 minutes

Cooking Time: 0 minutes

Servings: 2

Ingredients:

- ½ cup mixed berries (blueberries, strawberries, blackberries)
- 1 tablespoon ground flaxseed
- 2 tablespoons unsweetened coconut flakes
- ½ cup unsweetened plain coconut milk
- ½ cup leafy greens (kale, spinach)
- ¼ cup unsweetened vanilla nonfat yogurt
- ½ cup ice

Directions:

1. In a blender jar, combine the berries, flaxseed, coconut flakes, coconut milk, greens, yogurt, and ice.
2. Process until smooth. Serve.

Nutrition:

- Calories: 182 kcal
- Fat: 14.9g
- Carbohydrates: 8.1g
- Fiber: 4.1g
- Sugar: 2.9g
- Sodium: 25mg
- Protein: 5.9g

50. Walnut and Oat Granola

Preparation Time: 10 minutes

Cooking Time: 30 minutes

Servings: 8 granola bars

Ingredients:

- 2 cups rolled oats
- ½ cup walnut pieces
- ¼ cup pepitas
- ⅛ teaspoon salt
- ½ teaspoon ground cinnamon
- ½ teaspoon ground ginger
- ¼ cup coconut oil, melted
- ¼ cup unsweetened applesauce
- ½ teaspoon vanilla extract
- ¼ cup dried cherries

Directions:

1. The oven is set to 350°F (180°C) as preheating temperature. A baking sheet is prepared by lining it with parchment paper.
2. In a large bowl, toss the oats, walnuts, pepitas, salt, cinnamon, and ginger.
3. In a large measuring cup, combine the coconut oil, applesauce, and vanilla. Pour over the dry mixture and mix well.
4. Transfer the mixture to the parchment paper-lined baking sheet. Cook for 30 minutes, stirring about halfway through. Remove from the oven and let the granola sit undisturbed until completely cool. Break the granola into pieces, and stir in the dried cherries.
5. Transfer to an airtight container, and store at room temperature for up to 2 weeks.

Nutrition:

- Calories: 225 kcal
- Fat: 14.9g
- Carbohydrates: 20.1g
- Fiber: 3.1g
- Sugar: 4.9g

- Sodium: 31mg
- Protein: 4.9g

Snack

51. Easy Cauliflower Hush Puppies

Preparation Time: 15 minutes

Cooking Time: 10 minutes

Servings: 8 hush puppies

Ingredients:

- 1 whole cauliflower, including stalks and florets, roughly chopped
- ¾ cup buttermilk
- ¾ cup low-fat milk
- 1 medium onion, chopped
- 2 medium eggs
- 2 cups yellow cornmeal
- 1½ teaspoons baking powder
- ½ teaspoon salt

Directions:

1. In a blender, combine the cauliflower, buttermilk, milk, and onion and purée. Transfer to a large mixing bowl.
2. Crack the eggs into the purée, and gently fold until mixed.
3. In a medium bowl, whisk the cornmeal, baking powder, and salt together.
4. Gently add the dry ingredients to the wet ingredients and mix until just combined, taking care not to overmix.
5. Working in batches, place ⅓-cup portions of the batter into the basket of an air fryer.
6. Set the air fryer to 390°F (199°C), close, and cook for 10 minutes. Transfer the hush puppies to a plate. Repeat until no batter remains.
7. Serve warm with greens.

Nutrition:

- Calories: 180 kcal
- Fat: 8.1g

- Carbohydrates: 27.9g
- Fiber: 6.1g
- Sugar: 11.0g
- Sodium: 251mg
- Protein: 4.1g

Lunch

52. Veggie Fajitas with Guacamole

Preparation Time: 10 minutes

Cooking Time: 15 minutes

Servings: 2

Ingredients:

For the Guacamole:

- 1 small avocado pitted and peeled
- ½ teaspoon freshly squeezed lime juice
- ⅛ teaspoon salt
- 4 cherry tomatoes, halved

For the Fajitas:

- ½ red bell pepper
- ½ green bell pepper
- ½ small white onion
- Avocado oil cooking spray
- ½ cup low-sodium black beans in a can, drained and rinsed
- ¼ teaspoon ground cumin
- ⅛ teaspoon chili powder
- ⅛ teaspoon garlic powder
- 2 (6-inch) yellow corn tortillas

Directions:

To Make the Guacamole

1. In a medium bowl, use a fork to mash the avocados with the lime juice and salt.
2. Gently stir in the cherry tomatoes.

To Make the Fajitas

1. Cut the red bell pepper, green bell pepper, and onion into ½-inch slices.
2. Heat a large skillet over medium heat. When hot, coat the cooking surface with cooking spray. Put the peppers, onion, and beans into the skillet.
3. Add the cumin, chili powder, and garlic powder, and stir.
4. Cover and cook for 15 minutes, stirring halfway through.
5. Divide the fajita mixture equally between the tortillas, and top with guacamole and any preferred garnishes.

Nutrition:

- Calories: 270 kcal
- Fat: 15.1g
- Carbohydrates: 29.9g
- Fiber: 11.1g
- Sugar: 5.0g
- Sodium: 176mg

53. Spaghetti Squash and Chickpea Bolognese

Preparation Time: 5 minutes

Cooking Time: 25 minutes

Servings: 2

Ingredients:

- 1 (1 to 2-pound / 0.7- to 0.9-kg) spaghetti squash
- ¼ teaspoon ground cumin
- ½ cup no-sugar-added spaghetti sauce
- ½ (15 oz. / 425-g) can low-sodium chickpeas, drained and rinsed
- 3 oz. (80 g) extra-firm tofu

Directions:

1. The oven is set to pre-heating at 400°F (205°C).
2. Cut the squash in half lengthwise. Scoop out the seeds and discard.
3. Season both halves of the squash with the cumin, and place them on a baking sheet cut-side down. Roast for 25 minutes.
4. Meanwhile, heat a medium saucepan over low heat, and pour in the spaghetti sauce and chickpeas.
5. Wring out any excess water from the tofu using two layers of paper towels.
6. Crumble the tofu into the sauce and cook for 15 minutes.
7. Remove the squash from the oven, and comb through the flesh of each half with a fork to make thin strands.
8. Divide the "spaghetti" into four portions, and top each portion with one-quarter of the sauce.

Nutrition:

- Calories: 276 kcal
- Fat: 17.1g
- Carbohydrates: 41.9g
- Fiber: 10.1g
- Sugar: 7.0g
- Sodium: 56mg

Snack

54. Cauliflower Mash

Preparation Time: 7 minutes

Cooking Time: 20 minutes

Servings: 2

Ingredients:

- ½ head cauliflower, cored and cut into large florets
- ¼ teaspoon kosher salt
- ¼ teaspoon garlic pepper
- 1 tablespoon plain Greek yogurt
- Freshly grated Parmesan cheese
- ½ tablespoon unsalted butter or ghee (optional)
- Chopped fresh chives

Directions:

1. Pour 1 cup of water into the electric pressure cooker and insert a steamer basket or wire rack.
2. Place the cauliflower in the basket.
3. Secure the pressure cooker lid. Set the valve to sealing.
4. Cook on high pressure for 5 minutes.
5. When it beeps, hit Cancel and quickly release the pressure.
6. Remove the cauliflower from the pot and pour out the water. Return the cauliflower to the pot and add the salt, garlic pepper, yogurt, and cheese. Use an immersion blender or potato masher to purée or mash the cauliflower in the pot.
7. Spoon into a serving bowl, and garnish with butter (if using) and chives.

Nutrition:

- Calories: 141 kcal
- Fat: 6.1g
- Protein: 12.1g
- Carbohydrates: 11.9g

- Fiber: 4.1g
- Sugar: 5.0g
- Sodium: 591mg

Dinner

55. Chimichurri Dumplings

Preparation Time: 20 minutes

Cooking Time: 15 minutes

Servings: 2

Ingredients:

- 1 cup water
- 1 cup low-sodium vegetable broth
- ¼ cup cassava flour
- ¼ cup gluten-free all-purpose flour
- ½ teaspoons baking powder
- ¼ teaspoon salt
- ¼ cup fat-free milk
- ½ tablespoon bottled chimichurri or sofrito

Directions:

1. In a large pot, bring the water and the broth to a slow boil over medium-high heat.
2. In a large mixing bowl, whisk the cassava flour, all-purpose flour, baking powder, and salt together.
3. In a small bowl, whisk the milk and chimichurri together until combined.
4. Combine the wet ingredients into the dry ingredients a little at a time to create a firm dough.
5. With clean hands, pinch off a small piece of dough. Roll into a ball, and gently flatten in the palm of your hand, forming a disk. Repeat until no dough remains.
6. Carefully drop the dumplings one at a time into the boiling liquid. Cover and simmer for 15 minutes, or until the dumplings are cooked through. Inserting a fork into the dumpling should come out clean in order to judge that it is cooked.
7. Serve warm.

Nutrition:

- Calories: 133 kcal
- Fat: 1.1g
- Protein: 4.1g
- Carbohydrates: 25.9g
- Fiber: 3.1g
- Sugar: 2.0g
- Sodium: 328mg

56. Redux Okra Callaloo

Preparation Time: 15 minutes

Cooking Time: 25 minutes

Servings: 2

Ingredients:

- 1 cup low-sodium vegetable broth
- ⅓ (13.5 oz. / 383-g) can light coconut milk
- Coconut cream
- ⅓ tablespoon unsalted non-hydrogenated plant-based butter
- 4 oz. (110 g) okra, cut into 1-inch chunks
- ⅓ small onion, chopped
- Butternut squash, peeled, seeded, and cut into 4-inch chunks
- ⅓ bunch collard greens, stemmed and chopped
- ⅓ hot pepper (Scotch bonnet or habanero)

Directions:

1. In an electric pressure cooker, combine the vegetable broth, coconut milk, coconut cream, and butter.
2. Layer the okra, onion, squash, collard greens, and whole hot pepper on top.
3. Secure the lid, and set the pressure valve to sealing.
4. Select the Manual/Pressure Cook setting, and cook for 20 minutes.
5. Once cooking is complete, quick-release the pressure. Carefully remove the lid.
6. Remove and discard the hot pepper. Carefully transfer the callaloo to a blender, and blend until smooth. Serve spooned over grits.

Nutrition:

- Calories: 174 kcal
- Fat: 8.1g
- Protein: 4.1g
- Carbohydrates: 24.9g
- Fiber: 5.1g
- Sugar: 10.0g
- Sodium: 126mg

Chapter 14. Week 4 Meal Plan: Vegetarian and Weekly Shopping List

Breakfast

57. Coconut and Chia Pudding

Preparation Time: 5 minutes

Cooking Time: 0 minutes

Servings: 2

Ingredients:

- 7 oz. (198 g) light coconut milk
- ¼ cup chia seeds
- 3 to 4 drops liquid stevia
- 1 clementine
- 1 kiwi
- Shredded coconut (unsweetened)

Directions:

1. Start by taking a mixing bowl and adding in the light coconut milk. Add in the liquid stevia to sweeten the milk. Mix well.
2. Add the chia seeds to the milk and whisk until well-combined. Set aside.
3. Peel the clementine and carefully remove the skin from the wedges. Set aside.
4. Also, peel the kiwi and dice it into small pieces.
5. Take a glass jar and assemble the pudding. For this, place the fruits at the bottom of the jar; then add a dollop of chia pudding. Now spread the fruits and then add another layer of chia pudding.
6. Finish by garnishing with the remaining fruits and shredded coconut.

Nutrition:

- Calories: 486 kcal
- Fat: 40.5g
- Protein: 8.5g
- Carbohydrates: 30.8g
- Fiber: 15.6g
- Sugar: 11.6g
- Sodium: 24mg

58. Cottage Pancakes

Preparation Time: 10 minutes

Cooking Time: 20 minutes

Servings: 2

Ingredients:

- 1 cup low-fat cottage cheese
- 2 egg whites
- 1 egg
- ½ tablespoon pure vanilla extract
- ¾ cup almond flour
- Nonstick cooking spray

Directions:

1. Place the cottage cheese, egg whites, egg, and vanilla in a blender and pulse to combine.
2. The almond flour is added to the blender and blended until smooth.
3. Place a large nonstick skillet over medium heat and lightly coat it with cooking spray.
4. Spoon ¼ cup of batter per pancake, 4 at a time, into the skillet. Cook the pancakes until the bottoms are firm and golden, about 4 minutes.
5. Flip the pancakes to be able to cook the other side until they are cooked through, about 3 minutes.
6. Remove the pancakes to a plate and repeat with the remaining batter.
7. Serve with fresh fruit.

Nutrition:

- Calories: 345 kcal
- Fat: 22.1g
- Protein: 29.1g
- Carbohydrates: 11.1g
- Fiber: 4.1g
- Sugar: 5.1g
- Sodium: 560mg

Snack

59. Red Pepper, Goat Cheese, and Arugula Open-Faced Grilled Sandwich

Preparation Time: 5 minutes

Cooking Time: 15 minutes

Servings: 2

Ingredients:

- 1 red bell pepper, seeded
- Nonstick cooking spray
- 2 slice whole-wheat thin-sliced bread
- 4 tablespoons crumbled goat cheese
- Pinch dried thyme
- 1 cup arugula

Directions:

1. Preheat the broiler to high heat. Line a baking sheet with parchment paper.
2. Cut the ½ bell pepper lengthwise into two pieces and arrange on the prepared baking sheet with the skin facing up.
3. Broil until the skin is blackened for about 5 to 10 minutes. Transfer to a covered container to steam for 5 minutes, then remove the skin from the pepper using your fingers. Cut the pepper into strips.
4. Heat a small skillet over medium-high heat. Spray it with nonstick cooking spray and place the bread in the skillet. Top with the goat cheese and sprinkle with the thyme. Pile the arugula on top, followed by the roasted red pepper strips. Press down with a spatula to hold in place.
5. Cook for 2 to 3 minutes until the bread is crisp and browned and the cheese is warmed through. (If you prefer, you can make a half-closed sandwich instead: Cut the bread in half and place one half in the skillet. Top with the cheese, thyme, arugula, red pepper, and the other half slice of bread. Cook for 4 to 6 minutes, flipping once, until both sides are browned.)

Nutrition:

- Calories: 109 kcal
- Fat: 2g
- Protein: 4g
- Carbohydrates: 21g
- Fiber: 6g
- Sugar: 5g
- Sodium: 123mg

Lunch

60. Beet, Goat Cheese, and Walnut Pesto with Zoodles

Preparation Time: 15 minutes

Cooking Time: 40 minutes

Servings: 2

Ingredients:

- 1 medium red beet, peeled, chopped
- ½ cup walnut pieces
- 3 garlic cloves
- ½ cup crumbled goat cheese
- 2 tablespoons olive oil, plus 2 teaspoons
- 2 tablespoons freshly squeezed lemon juice
- ¼ teaspoon salt
- 4 small zucchinis

Directions:

1. Preheat the oven to 375°F.
2. Wrap the chopped beet in a piece of aluminum foil and seal well. Roast for 30 to 40 minutes until fork-tender.
3. Meanwhile, heat a dry skillet over medium-high heat. Toast the walnuts for 5 to 7 minutes until lightly browned and fragrant.
4. Transfer the cooked beets to the bowl of a food processor. Add the toasted walnuts, garlic, goat cheese, 2 tablespoons of olive oil, lemon juice, and salt. Process until smooth.
5. Using a spiralizer or sharp knife, cut the zucchini into thin "noodles."
6. Heat the remaining 2 teaspoons of oil over medium heat in a large skillet. Add the zucchini and toss in the oil. Cook, stirring gently, for 2 to 3 minutes, until the zucchini softens. Toss with the beet pesto and serve warm.

Nutrition:

- Calories: 422 kcal

- Total Fat: 39g
- Protein: 8g
- Carbohydrates: 17g
- Fiber: 6g
- Sugar: 10g
- Sodium: 339mg

61. Mushroom and Pesto Flatbread Pizza

Preparation Time: 5 minutes

Cooking Time: 15 minutes

Servings: 2

Ingredients:

- 1 teaspoon extra-virgin olive oil
- ½ cup sliced mushrooms
- ½ red onion, sliced
- Salt
- Freshly ground black pepper
- ¼ cup store-bought pesto sauce
- 2 whole-wheat flatbreads
- ¼ cup shredded mozzarella cheese

Directions:

1. Preheat the oven to 350°F.
2. Heat the oil in a small skillet. Add the mushrooms and onion, and season with salt and pepper. Sauté for 3 to 5 minutes until the onion and mushrooms begin to soften.
3. Spread 2 tablespoons of pesto on each flatbread.
4. Divide the mushroom-onion mixture between the two flatbreads. Top each with 2 tablespoons of cheese.
5. Bake the flatbreads for 10 to 12 minutes until the cheese is melted and bubbly. Serve warm.

Nutrition:

- Calories: 347 kcal
- Total Fat: 23g
- Protein: 14g
- Carbohydrates: 28g
- Fiber: 7g
- Sugar: 4g
- Sodium: 791mg

Snack

62. Cucumber, Tomato, and Avocado Salad

Preparation Time: 10 minutes

Cooking Time: 0 minutes

Servings: 2

Ingredients:

- ½ cup cherry tomatoes, halved
- 1 medium cucumber, chopped
- ½ small red onion, thinly sliced
- ½ avocado, diced
- 1 tablespoon chopped fresh dill
- 1 tablespoon extra-virgin olive oil
- Juice of ½ lemon
- ⅛ teaspoon salt
- ⅛ teaspoon freshly ground black pepper

Directions:

1. Combine the tomatoes, cucumber, onion, avocado, and dill in a large mixing bowl.
2. In a small bowl, combine the oil, lemon juice, salt, and pepper, and mix well.
3. Drizzle the dressing over the vegetables and toss to combine.
4. Serve.

Nutrition:

- Calories: 151 kcal
- Total Fat: 12g
- Protein: 2g
- Carbohydrates: 11g
- Fiber: 4g
- Sugar: 4g
- Sodium: 128mg

Dinner

63. Black Bean Enchilada Skillet Casserole

Preparation Time: 15 minutes

Cooking Time: 15 minutes

Servings: 2

Ingredients:

- ⅓ tablespoon extra-virgin olive oil
- Onion, chopped
- Red bell pepper, seeded and chopped
- Green bell pepper, seeded and chopped
- ⅔ small zucchini, chopped
- 1 garlic clove, minced
- ⅓ (15 oz.) can low-sodium black beans, drained and rinsed
- ⅓ (10 oz.) can low-sodium enchilada sauce
- ⅓ teaspoon ground cumin
- Salt
- Freshly ground black pepper
- Shredded cheddar cheese, divided
- ⅔ (6-inch) corn tortillas, cut into strips
- Chopped fresh cilantro, for garnish
- Plain yogurt, for serving

Directions:

1. Heat the broiler to high heat.
2. Pour some oil into a large oven-safe skillet.
3. Add the onion, red bell pepper, green bell pepper, zucchini, and garlic to the skillet, and cook for 3 to 5 minutes until the onion softens.
4. Add the black beans, enchilada sauce, cumin, salt, pepper, ¼ cup of cheese, and tortilla strips, and mix together. Top with the remaining ¼ cup of cheese.
5. Broil until you can see the cheese is melted and bubbly. Garnish with cilantro and serve with yogurt on the side.

Nutrition:

- Calories: 171 kcal
- Total Fat: 7g
- Protein: 8g
- Carbohydrates: 21g
- Fiber: 7g
- Sugar: 3g
- Sodium: 565mg

64. Crispy Parmesan Cups with White Beans and Veggies

Preparation Time: 10 minutes

Cooking Time: 5 minutes

Servings: 2

Ingredients:

- ½ cup grated Parmesan cheese, divided
- ½ (15 oz.) can low-sodium white beans, drained and rinsed
- ½ cucumber, peeled and finely diced
- ¼ cup finely diced red onion
- ⅛ cup thinly sliced fresh basil
- ½ garlic clove, minced
- ¼ jalapeño pepper, diced
- ½ tablespoon extra-virgin olive oil
- ½ tablespoon balsamic vinegar
- ⅛ teaspoon salt
- Freshly ground black pepper

Directions:

1. Sprinkle 2 tablespoons of cheese in a medium nonstick skillet and arrange it in a thin circle in the center of the pan, flattening it with a spatula.

2. When the cheese melts, use a spatula to flip the cheese and lightly brown the other side.

3. Remove the cheese "pancake" from the pan and place it into the cup of a muffin tin, bending it gently with your hands to fit in the muffin cup.

4. In a mixing bowl, combine the beans, cucumber, onion, basil, garlic, jalapeño, olive oil, and vinegar, and season with salt and pepper.

5. Fill each cup with the bean mixture just before serving.

Nutrition:

- Calories: 259 kcal
- Total Fat: 12g

- Protein: 15g
- Carbohydrates: 24g
- Fiber: 8g
- Sugar: 4g
- Sodium: 551mg

Chapter 15. Bonus: Sauces and Desserts Recipes

65. Fruit-and-nut-stuffed Baked Apples

Preparation Time: 5 minutes

Cooking Time: 50 minutes

Servings: 2

Ingredients:

- ½ teaspoon canola oil
- ¼ cup dried cranberries
- 1 tablespoon chopped walnuts
- ¼ teaspoon ground cinnamon
- 2 medium Granny Smith or Rome apples
- ¼ cup apple cider
- ¼ cup water
- 1 teaspoon unbleached all-purpose flour

Directions:

1. Preheat the oven to 350°F. Spray oil into an 8-inch square glass baking dish.
2. Combine the cranberries, walnuts, and cinnamon in a small bowl and toss to coat. Set aside.
3. Core the apples, taking time to cut to the bottoms, but not through. Cut away 1 inch of the peel from the tops of the apples. Divide the cranberry mixture evenly among the apples, pressing the mixture into each cavity. Arrange the apples upright in the prepared baking dish.
4. Combine the apple cider, water, and flour in a medium bowl and whisk until smooth. Pour over the apples.
5. Bake, uncovered, basting twice, until the apples are tender, 40 to 45 minutes.
6. To serve, place the apples in shallow bowls and drizzle evenly with the sauce. Serve hot, warm, or at room temperature.

Nutrition:

- Carbohydrates: 37g
- Calories: 175 kcal
- Fat: 4g
- Saturated Fat: 0g
- Cholesterol: 0mg
- Fiber: 5g
- Protein: 1g
- Sodium: 5mg

66. Creamy Custard Sauce

Preparation Time: 5 minutes

Cooking Time: 10 minutes

Servings: 2

Ingredients:

- ½ cup 1% low-fat milk
- 1 small egg yolks
- Sugar
- Cornstarch
- Pinch of salt
- Vanilla extract

Directions:

1. Combine the milk, egg yolks, sugar, cornstarch, and salt in a medium saucepan. Cook until the sauce boils and thickens, about 5 minutes taking care to stir frequently.
2. Turn off the heat and whisk in the vanilla. Pour into a serving bowl and let cool slightly to serve warm. To serve chilled, place a sheet of wax paper on the surface of the sauce to prevent a skin from forming. Let the sauce cool to room temperature. The sauce can be stored in the refrigerator for up to 3 days.

Nutrition:

- Carbohydrates: 9g
- Calories: 53 kcal
- Fat: 1g
- Saturated Fat: 1g
- Cholesterol: 42mg
- Fiber: 0g
- Protein: 2g
- Sodium: 30mg

67. Orange and Pink Grapefruit Salad with Honey-rosemary Syrup

Preparation Time: 5 minutes

Cooking Time: 40 minutes

Servings: 2

Ingredients:

- 1 tablespoon honey
- 1 tablespoon orange juice
- 1 teaspoon fresh rosemary leaves
- 1 large navel oranges
- ½ large pink grapefruit

Directions:

1. Combine the honey, orange juice, and rosemary in a small saucepan. Bring to a boil over medium heat. Let stand 30 minutes to cool. Pour through a fine wire-mesh strainer into a small bowl. Discard the rosemary.
2. Meanwhile, cut a thin slice from the top and bottom of the oranges and the grapefruit, exposing the flesh. Stand each fruit upright, and using a sharp knife, thickly cut off the peel, following the contour of the fruit and removing all the white pith and membrane. Thinly slice the fruit into rounds.
3. To serve, layer the grapefruit and orange slices alternately on a serving platter and drizzle with the syrup.

Nutrition:

- Carbohydrates: 25g
- Calories: 96 kcal
- Fat: 0g
- Saturated Fat: 0g
- Cholesterol: 0mg
- Fiber: 2g
- Protein: 1g
- Sodium: 1mg

68. Fruit-filled Meringues with Custard Sauce

Preparation Time: 5 minutes

Cooking Time: 40 minutes

Servings: 2

Ingredients:

- ⅔ large ripe kiwi, peeled and chopped
- ⅓ cup quartered fresh strawberries
- ⅓ cup fresh blueberries

Directions:

1. Prepare Meringue Cookies according to the instructions, but place the beaten egg white mixture on the prepared pan and use the back of a spoon to spread it into six 4-inch circles, creating indentations in the center of each one. Proceed with the recipe as directed.
2. Combine the kiwi, strawberries, and blueberries in a medium bowl and toss to mix well.
3. To assemble, place a baked meringue on each of 6 plates. Top each meringue with about ½ cup of the fruit mixture. Drizzle evenly with the sauce and serve at once.

Nutrition:

- Carbohydrates: 39g
- Calories: 194 kcal
- Fat: 2g
- Saturated Fat: 1g
- Cholesterol: 71mg
- Fiber: 2g
- Protein: 5g
- Sodium: 79mg

69. Frozen Yogurt

Preparation Time: 5 minutes

Cooking Time: 5 minutes plus up to 2 hours' refrigeration time

Servings: 2

Ingredients:

- ¼ cup 1% low-fat milk
- Sugar
- ¼ cup plain low-fat yogurt
- Vanilla extract

Directions:

1. In a small saucepan, combine milk and sugar. Stirring often, until the sugar dissolves, cook over medium heat, about 3 minutes (do not boil). Transfer to a small bowl and let cool to room temperature. Refrigerate, covered, until chilled, about 2 hours.
2. Whisk together the milk mixture, yogurt, and vanilla in a medium bowl until smooth. Transfer the mixture into an ice cream maker and let it freeze. Transfer to an airtight container and freeze overnight. The yogurt can be frozen, covered, for up to 1 week.

Nutrition:

- Carbohydrates: 25g
- Calories: 125 kcal
- Fat: 1g
- Saturated Fat: 1g
- Cholesterol: 5mg
- Fiber: 0g
- Protein: 4g
- Sodium: 56mg

70. Peach-blueberry Crostata

Preparation Time: 5 minutes

Cooking Time: 40 minutes

Servings: 2 (6 crostatas each)

Ingredients:

- 1 recipe Pastry Crust
- 1 lb. peaches, peeled, pitted, and sliced (about 3 cups)
- ½ cup fresh blueberries or unthawed frozen blueberries
- ¼ cup plus 2 teaspoons sugar, divided
- ¼ cup unbleached all-purpose flour
- 1 teaspoon grated lemon zest
- ¼ teaspoon ground cinnamon
- 2 teaspoons unsalted butter, melted

Directions:

1. Preheat the oven to 400°F.
2. Arrange the pastry dough between two sheets of parchment paper. Roll the dough into a 12-inch circle. Set aside, leaving the dough between the parchment paper to prevent it from drying out.
3. Combine the peaches, blueberries, ¼ cup of the sugar, the flour, lemon zest, and cinnamon in a large bowl and toss to coat. Transfer the dough inside the parchment paper sheets onto a large baking sheet. Remove the top layer of parchment.
4. The fruit mixture is placed in a mound in the center of the dough. Carefully fold the dough up and over the edge of the filling, pleating as necessary. Brush the dough with the melted butter and sprinkle with the remaining 2 teaspoons of sugar. Bake until the fruit is bubbly and the crust is browned, 30 to 35 minutes. Serve warm or at room temperature. The crostata is best the day it is made.

Nutrition:

- Carbohydrates: 27g
- Calories: 163 kcal
- Fat: 6g
- Saturated Fat: 3g

- Cholesterol: 14mg
- Fiber: 3g
- Protein: 2g
- Sodium: 59mg

71. Creamy Goat Cheese—chive Dressing

Preparation Time: 5 minutes

Cooking Time: 0 minutes

Servings: 2 (¼ cup each)

Ingredients:

- ½ cup plain low-fat yogurt
- 2 tablespoons mayonnaise
- 2 tablespoons finely crumbled soft goat cheese
- 1 teaspoon white wine vinegar
- 1 small garlic clove, crushed
- ¼ teaspoon kosher salt
- ⅛ teaspoon freshly ground pepper
- 2 tablespoons minced fresh chives

Directions:

1. In a small bowl, whisk together all the ingredients. Stir in the chives. The dressing can be refrigerated, covered, for up to 3 days.

Nutrition:

- Carbohydrates: 1g
- Calories: 42 kcal
- Fat: 4g
- Saturated Fat: 1g
- Cholesterol: 4mg
- Fiber: 0g
- Protein: 1g
- Sodium: 74mg

72. Pecan Pie

Preparation Time: 5 minutes

Cooking Time: 50 minutes

Servings: 2 (6 pies each)

Ingredients:

- 1 recipe Pastry Crust
- ¾ cup light corn syrup
- ½ cup packed light brown sugar
- 2 large eggs
- 1 large egg white
- 3 tablespoons unbleached all-purpose flour
- 1 tablespoon unsalted butter, melted
- 1 teaspoon vanilla extract
- Pinch of salt
- ¾ cup pecans, toasted and coarsely chopped

Directions:

1. Preheat the oven to 350°F.
2. Arrange the pastry dough between two sheets of wax paper. Roll the dough into a 12-inch circle. Remove the top layer of wax paper and place the dough, with the wax paper facing up, into a 9-inch glass pie plate. Starting from the edge of the dough, gently remove the wax paper. Crimp the edge decoratively.
3. Whisk together the corn syrup, sugar, eggs, egg white, flour, butter, vanilla, and salt in a medium bowl until smooth. Stir in the pecans. Pour the filling into the prepared crust. Bake until the crust is browned and the filling is almost set, for about 40 to 45 minutes.
4. Let the pie cool completely on a wire rack before slicing. The pie is best the day it is made.

Nutrition:

- Carbohydrates: 38g
- Calories: 251 kcal
- Fat: 11g
- Saturated Fat: 4g
- Cholesterol: 48mg

- Fiber: 2g
- Protein: 3g
- Sodium: 94mg

73. Panna Cotta

Preparation Time: 5 minutes

Cooking Time: 10 minutes

Servings: 2

Ingredients:

- ⅔ teaspoons canola oil
- 1 cup 2% low-fat milk, divided
- ⅓ tablespoon unflavored gelatin
- Sugar
- ⅓ tablespoon vanilla extract

Directions:

1. Brush two 6 oz. ramekins or custard cups with the oil.
2. Place 2 cups of the milk in a medium saucepan. Sprinkle with the gelatin and let stand 2 minutes to soften. Add the sugar and cook over medium heat, stirring constantly, until the mixture thickens and coats the back of a spoon (do not boil). Turn off the heat and add in the remaining 2 cups of milk and vanilla. Divide the mixture among the prepared ramekins. Refrigerate the custards, covered, overnight.
3. To serve, loosen the edge of each panna cotta with a knife and invert the ramekins onto individual plates.

Nutrition:

- Carbohydrates: 23g
- Calories: 149 kcal
- Fat: 4g
- Saturated Fat: 2g
- Cholesterol: 10mg
- Fiber: 0g
- Protein: 5g
- Sodium: 53mg

74. Tapioca Pudding

Preparation Time: 5 minutes

Cooking Time: 15 minutes

Servings: 2

Ingredients:

- 1 cup 1% low-fat milk
- ½ large egg
- Sugar
- 1 tablespoon minute tapioca
- Salt
- ½ teaspoon vanilla extract

Directions:

1. Combine the milk, egg, sugar, tapioca, and salt in a medium saucepan and stir to mix well. Let stand for 5 minutes.
2. Cook the milk mixture until the mixture comes to a boil, about 6 minutes. Turn off the heat and stir in the vanilla. Transfer the pudding to a medium bowl and place a sheet of wax paper on the surface of the pudding to prevent a skin from forming. Cool to room temperature. Stir the pudding and refrigerate, covered, until chilled, 4 hours or overnight.

Nutrition:

- Carbohydrates: 31g
- Calories: 173 kcal
- Fat: 2g
- Saturated Fat: 1g
- Cholesterol: 59mg
- Fiber: 0g
- Protein: 6g
- Sodium: 144mg

75. Balsamic Vinaigrette

Preparation Time: 5 minutes

Cooking Time: 0 minutes

Servings: 2 (⅙ cup each)

Ingredients:

- 3 tablespoons extra virgin olive oil
- 2 tablespoons balsamic vinegar
- 1 tablespoon minced shallots
- 1 teaspoon honey
- ½ teaspoon Dijon mustard
- ¼ teaspoon kosher salt
- ⅛ teaspoon freshly ground pepper

Directions:

1. Combine all the ingredients in a small bowl. The dressing can be refrigerated, covered, for up to 3 days.

Nutrition:

- Carbohydrates: 2g
- Calories: 54 kcal
- Fat: 5g
- Saturated Fat: 1g
- Cholesterol: 0mg
- Fiber: 0g
- Protein: 0g
- Sodium: 39mg

Conclusion

Why did I start this book? Having Type 1 diabetes will teach you a load of tough lessons. Only about ¼ of diabetics are Type 1. But I'm here to tell you, even though Type 1 is the most common type of diabetes, Type 2 diabetes can be almost as bad. I'm telling you this because I don't want you to get discouraged and give up.

Being diagnosed with the disease will bring some major changes in your lifestyle. From the time you are diagnosed with it, it would always be a constant battle with food. You need to become a lot more careful with your food choices and the quantity that you ate. Every meal will feel like a major effort. You will be planning every day for the whole week, well in advance. Depending upon the type of food you ate, you have to keep checking your blood sugar levels. You may get used to taking long breaks between meals and staying away from snacks between dinner and breakfast.

Food would be treated as a bomb like it can go off at any time. According to an old saying, "When the body gets too hot, then your body heads straight to the kitchen."

Managing diabetes can be a very, very stressful ordeal. There will be many times that you will mark your glucose levels down on a piece of paper like you are plotting graph lines or something. You will mix your insulin shots up and then stress about whether or not you are giving yourself the right dosage. You will always be over-cautious because it involves a LOT of math and a really fine margin of error. But now, those days are gone!

With the help of technology and books, you can stock your kitchen with the right foods, like meal plans, diabetic friendly dishes, etc. You can get an app that will even do the work for you. You can also people-watch on the internet and find the know-how to cook and eat right; you will always be a few meals away from certain disasters, like a plummeting blood sugar level. Always carry some sugar in your pocket. You won't have to experience the pangs of hunger but if you are unlucky, you will have to ration your food and bring along some simple low-calorie snacks with you.

This is the future of diabetes.

As you've reached the end of this book, you have gained complete control of your diabetes and this is just the beginning of your journey towards a better, healthier life. I hope I was able to inculcate some knowledge into you and make this adventure a little bit less of a struggle.

I would like to remind you that you're not alone in having to manage this disease and that nearly 85% of the new cases are 20 years old or younger.

Regardless of the length or seriousness of your diabetes, it can be managed! Take the information presented here and start with it!

Preparation is key to having a healthier and happier life.

It's helpful to remember that every tool at your disposal can help in some way.